HOMEOPATHY

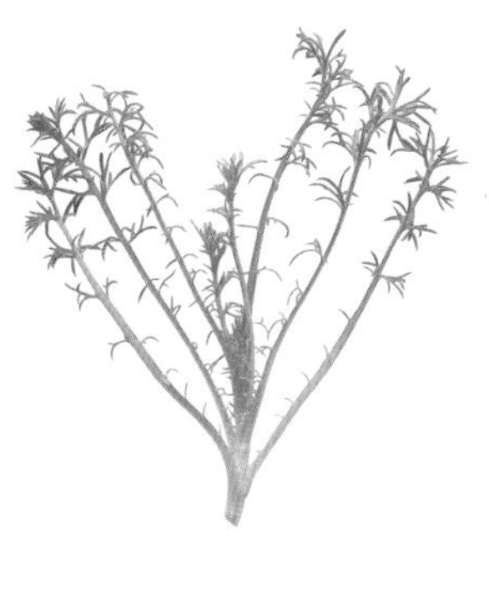

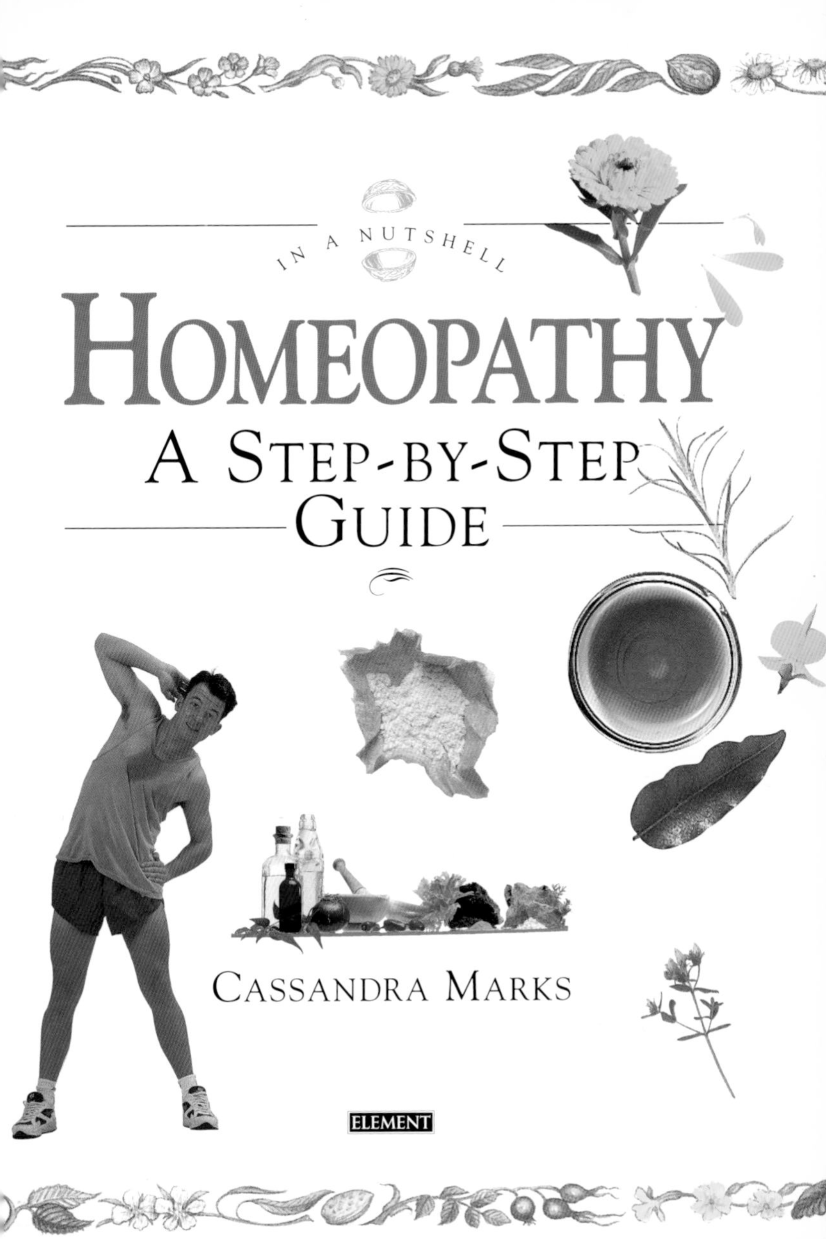

IN A NUTSHELL

HOMEOPATHY

A STEP-BY-STEP GUIDE

CASSANDRA MARKS

ELEMENT

This edition
published in 2002
by Element,
an Imprint of HarperCollins*Publishers*,
77-85 Fulham Palace Road,
London W6 8JB

The Element website address is:
www.elementbooks.co.uk

First published in Great Britain in 1997 by
ELEMENT BOOKS LIMITED

NOTE FROM THE PUBLISHER
Any information given in this book is not intended to be taken as a replacement for medical advice. Any person with a condition requiring medical attention should consult a qualified practitioner or therapist.

Designed and created with
The Bridgewater Book Company Limited

THE BRIDGEWATER BOOK COMPANY
Art Director Peter Bridgewater
Designers Andrew Milne, Jane Lanaway
Page layout Chris Lanaway, Sue Rose
Managing Editor Anne Townley
Picture Research Lynda Marshall
Three dimensional models Mark Jamieson
Photography Ian Parsons, Guy Ryecart
Illustrations Andrew Milne,
Andrew Kulman
Editorial consultants

Printed and bound in Hong Kong by Printing Express

British Library Cataloguing in
Publication data available

Library of Congress Cataloging in
Publication data available

ISBN 0-00-714041-X

The publishers wish to thank
the following for the use of pictures:
Harry Smith Collection: pp. 32L, 32TR;
The Homeopathic Trust: pp. 8TL, 9CL;
Janine Wiedel Photolibrary: pp. 35;
Science Photo Library: pp. 14B, 24R, 25,
29R, 31T, 37, 49

Special thanks go to:
Tom Aitken, Tony Bannister, Ian Clegg,
Eddie Cooper, Gail Downey, Carly Evans,
Julia Holden, Robin Yarnton
for help with photography

Steamer Trading Company,
Lewes, Sussex, UK
for help with properties

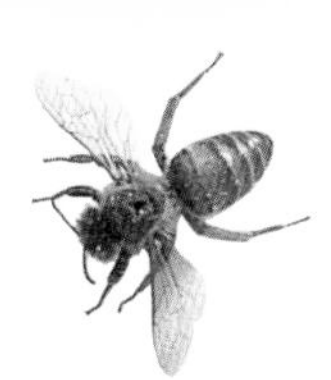

Contents

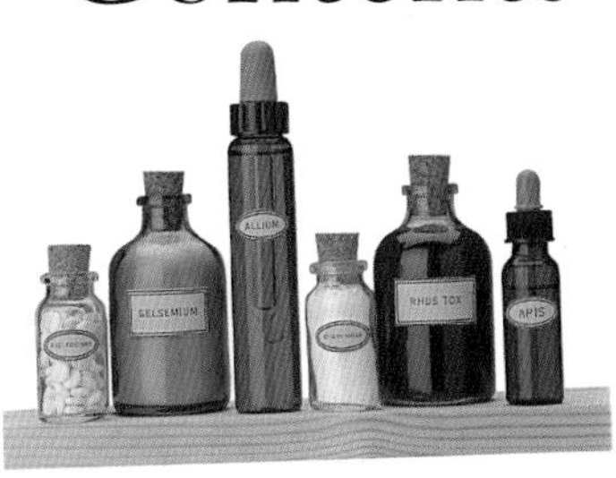

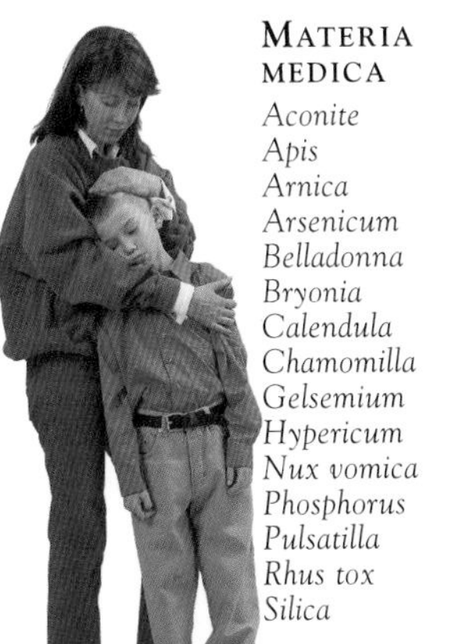

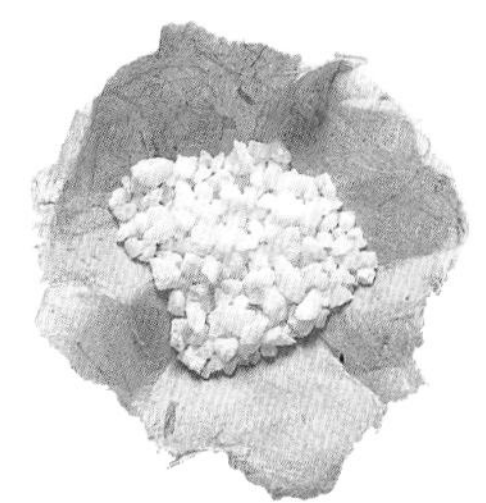

What is homeopathy?

HOMEOPATHY IS A NATURAL *system of medicine that uses specially prepared remedies to stimulate the immune system. Although some remedies are made from herbs, homeopathy shouldn't be confused with herbalism. Herbal remedies use material concentrations of plants, while homeopathic remedies use plants, minerals, and even some animal products as a base. They are prepared through a process known as "potentization" to bring out their subtle healing properties.*

Homeopathy is an "energy" system of medicine – based on a model of the human body which includes an energy field or "vital" force. We know from modern physics that our seemingly solid bodies are dense fields of energy. A disturbance in this field can give rise to disease, and a potent form of energy can rebalance us. Homeopathy uses "potentized" remedies to rebalance our body's subtle energy system. Once this is back in balance, our immune systems and all the other interconnected systems in our bodies start functioning better.

LEFT ***Minerals are ground with lactose, while plant-based remedies are prepared from tinctures (plants suspended in alcohol).***

The term "homeopathy" comes from the Greek, meaning "similar suffering." It reflects the key principle behind the homeopathic method – that a substance can cure the symptoms in an ill person that it is capable of causing in a healthy person.

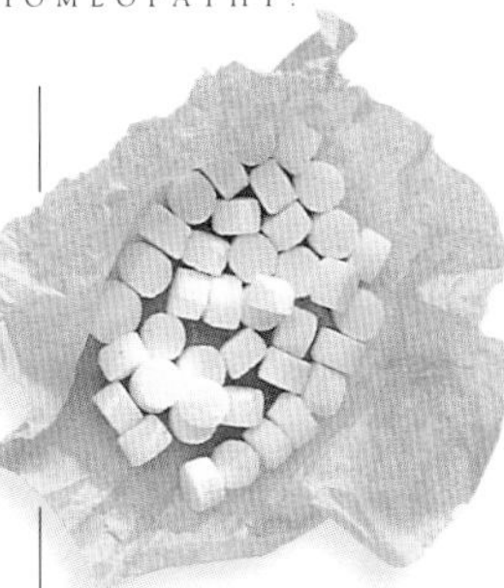

LEFT *Homeopathic remedies are prepared with milk sugar. They taste sweet and dissolve quickly.*

LEFT *Health is more than a matter of appearances. It's about an inner vitality and a sense of well-being.*

WHY USE HOMEOPATHY?

No homeopathic remedies are tested on animals. Because they've all been tested on healthy people, we know their effect on the human body. In acute illness homeopathy:

- Treats acute symptoms safely and effectively
- Has no side-effects
- Works with the immune system rather than against it
- Improves resistance to infection
- Shortens recovery time after illness – often preventing complications

BELOW *Homeopathy uses subtle remedies to rebalance your energy.*

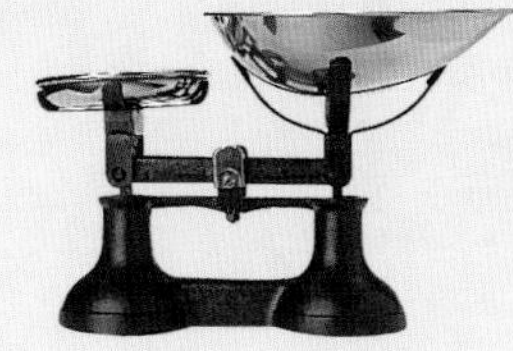

A short history

THE THERAPEUTIC PRINCIPLE *that "like cures like" keeps cropping up in medical literature, at least since the time of the healer and "father of medicine," Hippocrates (around 100* B.C.*).*

ABOVE ***The founder of homeopathy, Dr. Samuel Hahnemann (1755–1843) lived and taught in Germany, later establishing a practice in Paris at the age of 79.***

It was Dr. Samuel Hahnemann who made this principle the foundation of a new system of medicine. Hahnemann was an 18th-century German physician who had become disillusioned with the side-effects of medical treatments.

While investigating the anti-malarial effects of cinchona bark (quinine), he discovered it gave him just that type of fever.

Between 1790 and 1805 Hahnemann tested 60 drugs from a variety of sources on himself and a small group of students. This method of "proving" substances to discover the range of symptoms they were capable of causing enabled Hahnemann to find out what they could also cure.

ABOVE ***Cinchona in homeopathic form; the remedy is called China.***

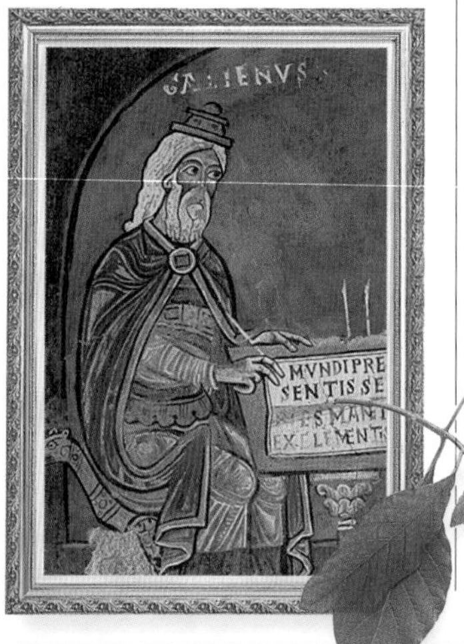

LEFT ***Leaves of the cinchona tree. The bark contains quinine, which was used for Hahnemann's first experiment.***

THE PRINCIPLES OF HOMEOPATHY

Symptoms caused by material doses

Ingesting the poisonous berries of deadly nightshade (the plant Belladonna) causes:

- Tight throat
- Difficulty swallowing
- Vomiting
- Delirium
- Coma and even death

Symptoms cured by homeopathic doses

In homeopathic form Belladonna cures:

- Infections with high fever and delirium (sufferer sees black shapes)
- Sore throat
- Thirst

RIGHT ***Deadly nightshade plant, used for Belladonna.***

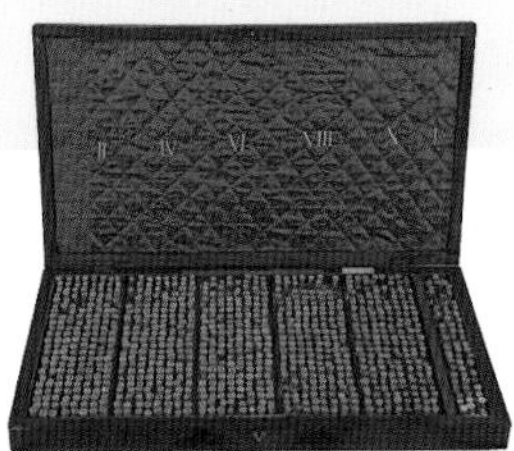

ABOVE ***Hahnemann used this wooden case to store hundreds of remedies.***

Later, homeopathic physicians tested or "proved" minerals such as sulfur, phosphorus, and quartz (Silica), as well as oyster shells (Calcarea carbonica), gold (Aurum), the honeybee (Apis), bushmaster snake venom (Lachesis), and plants such as foxglove (Digitalis) and the windflower (Pulsatilla). There are over 3,000 homeopathic remedies, which come from a range of sources.

In Hahnemann's time diseases were treated with large doses of toxic substances, and many patients were literally poisoned by such medicines as arsenic and mercury. Hahnemann was careful to test these substances for their homeopathic effects in a very dilute form. Paradoxically, he found that the effectiveness of the remedy actually increased as it became more dilute – doing away with the problem of side-effects at the same time. Hahnemann developed a system of successive dilution and "succussion," in which the remedy is shaken vigorously to release the healing potential in substances.

How does homeopathy work?

HOMEOPATHIC REMEDIES *stimulate our immune system to deal with disease more effectively. A homeopath will acknowledge all of your symptoms, including any emotional and mental changes, and with that information, make an assessment of your individual constitution and any imbalances. A remedy that will match your exact condition is then prescribed. Over the centuries, a sophisticated homeopathic model has been developed which allows us to understand how all our symptoms relate to each other. Homeopathy never treats symptoms alone, but attempts to find the underlying problem from which all of the symptoms stem. Modern immunology has a fancy term for this, calling it the "psycho-neuro-immunology" disturbance. In layman's terms, that means that only when your core problems are sorted out can your energy levels improve and your physical symptoms be cured.*

Homeopathic principles make a treatment homeopathic. What makes a medicine homeopathic is not just how it's made, but whether you use it according to these principles, which are:

- Like cures like. That which can cause disease can also cure it, by stimulating the body to defend itself against it.
- Minimum dose. You should take the least amount of medicine needed to get back on the right track.
- Law of cure. Obvious problems start to heal first, allowing underlying problems to surface that can then be treated as well.

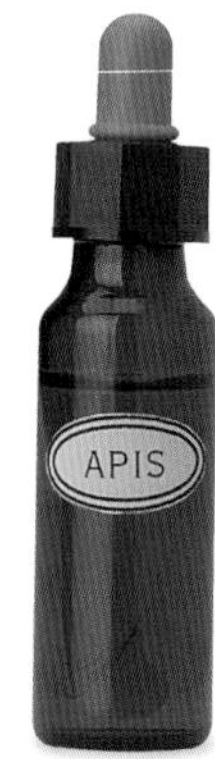

HOMEOPATHIC DILUTION

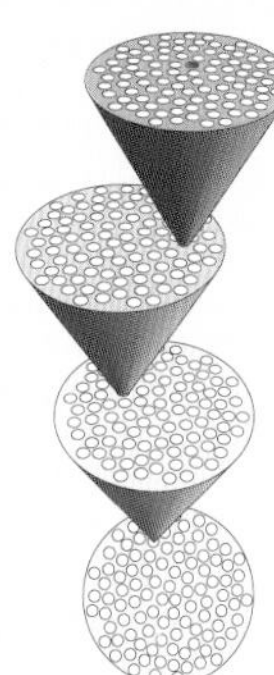

ABOVE **The higher the potency of the remedy, the more it has been diluted.**

Homeopathy uses preparations containing infinitesimal amounts of the original substance – whether from something poisonous like Belladonna or something innocuous like salt (Natrum mur). For example: to make the 6 potency (properly called the 6 centesimal potency) of Arsenicum album, one part of arsenic is added to 99 parts of milk sugar or alcohol and succussed, and this process is repeated 6 times. A 30 potency has gone through the same process 30 times. Although a 30 potency has been diluted more than the 6 potency, the succussion has made it more powerful and it is usually taken for more serious problems than a 6 potency. (The number on the label tells you just how many dilutions the remedy has been through.)

Remedies can also be diluted according to the decimal scale; that is, one part to nine. In this case, there will be an x next to the number – e.g., 6x.

THE LAW OF CURE

Homeopathy has developed a precise hierarchy of symptoms, with which to evaluate your overall level of health or illness. It is also valuable in signposting the road to recovery. Learning to understand the messages your body gives you will help you to be treated more successfully.

Symptoms should disappear in reverse order to their original appearance

Healing progresses from more important organs to less important ones

Healing progresses from the top of the body downward (especially in the case of skin rashes)

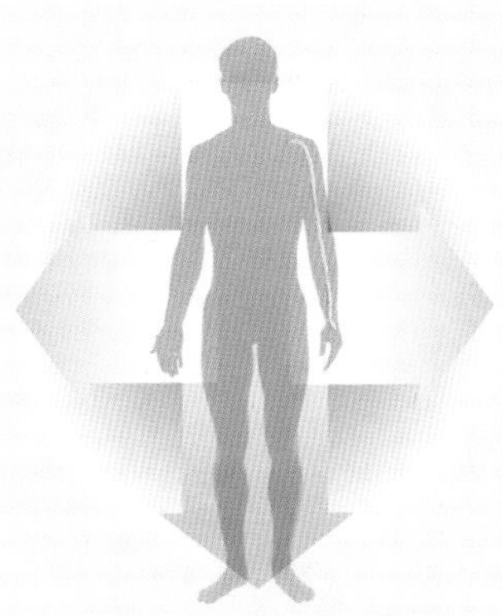

The body seeks to externalize disease – keeping it to more external locations

You can use this law to help you evaluate the success of any form of treatment you are receiving

How homeopathy views symptoms

CONVENTIONAL MEDICINE *treats symptoms rather than attempting to find the root problem. Treatment involves suppressing or wiping out the symptoms with drugs. But many common symptoms that we regard as signs of illness are actually positive signs of a healthy immune response. Fever and inflammation are the strategies the body uses to deal effectively with microbes.*

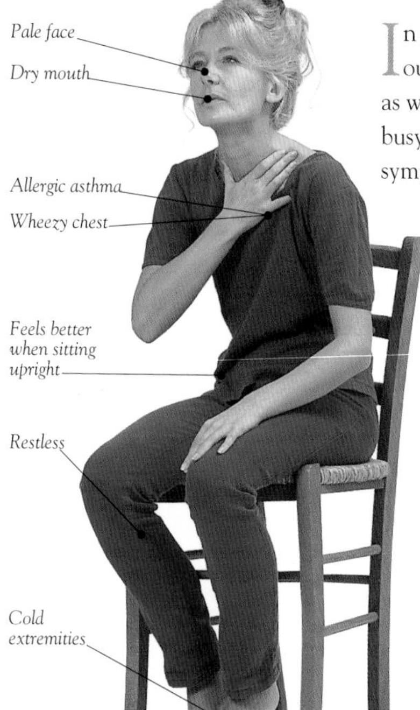

In response to acute infections, our bodies can clear out toxins, as well as taking a rest from a busy and stressful lifestyle. Mild symptoms are signs that the body is working efficiently to deal with illness, and when they are more serious, they indicate the areas where you need some support.

LEFT ***Detailed symptoms provide important clues in choosing a remedy. Some important indicators may include: temperature, feeling cold and shivery, yet wanting fresh air; runny nose; wheezing; thirst for cold water; desire for ice; physically restless; aching muscles; diarrhea (see Arsenicum, page 28).***

Severe symptoms are signs that your body is under stress, and needs treatments that support the efforts of the immune system. Symptoms are messages from the body, and we must learn to read them.

SOME COMMON REASONS TO VISIT A HOMEOPATH

- Effects of stress
- Post-traumatic stress syndrome
- Phobias
- Psychological problems and depression
- ME and glandular fever
- Hepatitis
- Epilepsy; allergies
- Repeated infections
- PMS
- Hormonal problems associated with periods, fertility, or menopause
- Acne
- Herpes
- Chronic thrush and cystitis
- Migraines
- Irritable bowel syndrome
- Colitis
- Arthritis
- Complaints associated with pregnancy
- To aid childbirth
- Infections and ailments of infants and children
- Behavioral problems
- Hyperactivity

Homeopathy can be used to treat almost any condition.

CASE HISTORIES

Sulfur

An adolescent boy came in complaining of allergies. He had suffered allergic rhinitis for several years, as well as eczema which erupted a few months after his childhood vaccinations. His skin was worse when he was too hot, especially in bed. He seemed hot all the time, with sweaty feet. Eggs and spicy foods aggravated his eczema. He sneezed a lot every morning, and his nose blocked up in the open air. Although bright, he was a bit of a loner, spending hours playing computer games. His personality and metabolism provided an important pointer to the choice of his remedy, in this case Sulfur.

SULFUR

Natrum mur

A woman of 44, suffering from migraines and depression, was treated with Natrum mur. The migraines came before each period, and had started after her son's death some years earlier. Since then she'd felt very depressed, often crying into the night. She'd become much more reclusive and sensitive. She became moody at the slightest criticism, and had gone off love-making. Her "core" problem was grief. The fact that grief had triggered her symptoms was important in helping the homeopath decide which remedy was right.

NATRUM MUR

Treatment

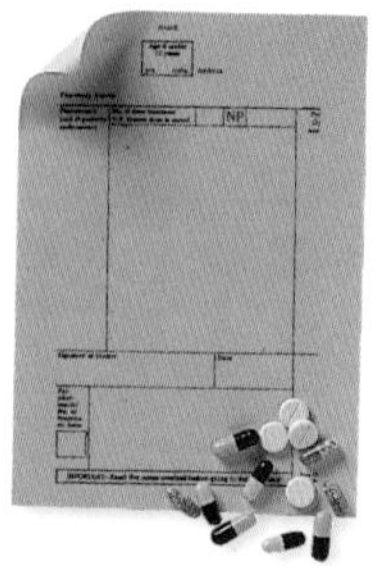

ABOVE **A homeopath will supply you with remedies, while a physician provides a prescription.**

HOMEOPATHS TREAT THE SAME *range of complaints as a general practitioner. In the hands of a skilled practitioner, homeopathy can treat psychological problems and serious chronic illnesses such as MS. Other examples of deeper problems are allergies (such as eczema, hay fever, and asthma), repeated infections of any nature, and depression or obsessional states.*

HOMEOPATHY AND COLDS

Homeopathic remedies are very good for treating infections and catarrhal problems, clearing up fevers, colds, coughs, sore throats, runny noses, and earaches quickly. If you're basically healthy, you should be able to throw off a cold with a couple of days of rest. However, whenever colds turn into prolonged coughs, affect the ears, or go down to the chest, your body needs help to deal with the infection. The conventional way of dealing with infection – giving antibiotics – is rarely justified. Antibiotics kill off friendly as well as harmful bacteria in the body, and since colds are caused by viruses, they are usually entirely inappropriate. Antibiotics also tend to make you more run down, leaving you open to further infection.

BELOW ***Many of the symptoms following infection are front-line immune responses. For example, a raised temperature encourages the immune system; a runny nose indicates that your body is producing mucus to wash out irritants; a cough is necessary to clear catarrh out of your airways.***

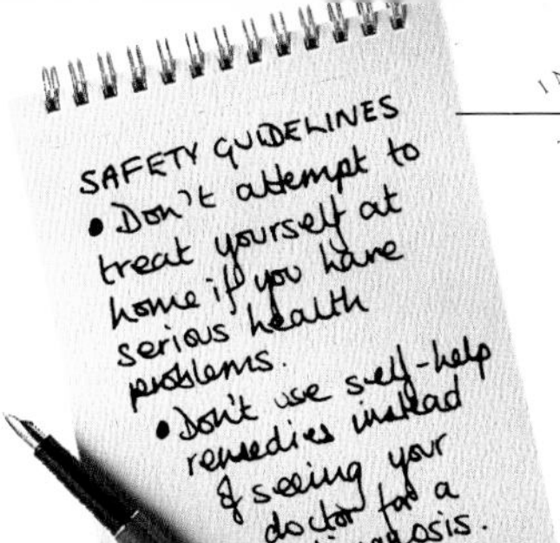

Homeopaths differentiate between acute illnesses – usually short illnesses that blow up quickly and blow over quickly as well – and more serious (chronic, or long-term) "constitutional" problems. In constitutional treatment a single homeopathic remedy is chosen to cover all your problems – both physical and psychological. Classical homeopaths, who practice according to traditional techniques, usually give just one high potency dose of a remedy, and carefully watch your response. If it's the correct remedy, this high potency stimulates your energy, improving your mood and sense of well-being, before balancing out your body systems. This type of prescribing is quite an art, and it takes several years to perfect.

This sort of constitutional treatment usually involves monthly sessions over several months – or even years, depending on how long you've been suffering from health problems.

BELOW ***Consulting a homeopath involves detailed questions about yourself. You often discover connections between your different problems.***

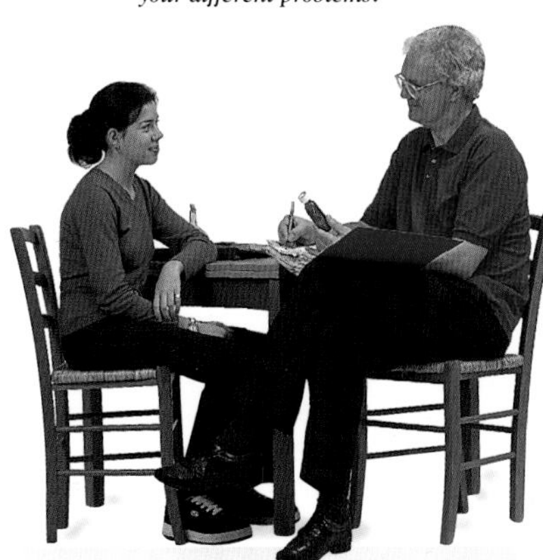

WHEN SHOULD I SEEK PROFESSIONAL ADVICE?

- Seek professional advice when self-help treatment isn't working
- If you are suffering from general stress and tiredness, with a lowered resistance to infections, or a range of minor health problems
- If your life feels badly out of balance, whether due to stress, emotional problems or physical complaints
- If you suffer from serious health problems of any nature

Homeopathic techniques

IF YOU GET THE HOMEOPATHIC *remedy right, it works quickly – especially in acute illnesses that come on quickly, such as infections. If you haven't chosen the right remedy, you can tell it's not working because there is no improvement in the symptoms. Homeopathy is as good as your ability to choose the right remedy. That involves carefully distinguishing between different remedy pictures.*

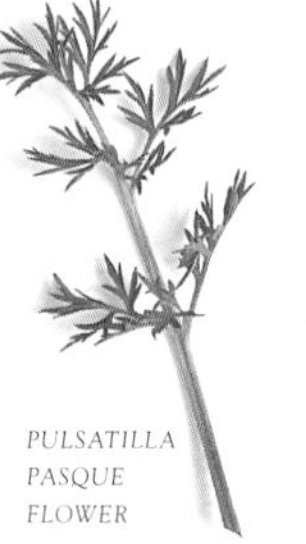
PULSATILLA PASQUE FLOWER

Symptoms are the key to choosing an appropriate homeopathic remedy, because they show exactly how the body is trying to restore balance. Clues to the right remedy are found in details such as the location and type of inflammation (e.g., whether in the throat, chest, or ears), or the kind of discharge produced (irritating mucus, creamy, or thick and yellow-green). The conditions that trigger off a particular infection (such as the damp, stress, or emotions) show the circumstances which lower our resistance to illness.

MIXING THERAPIES

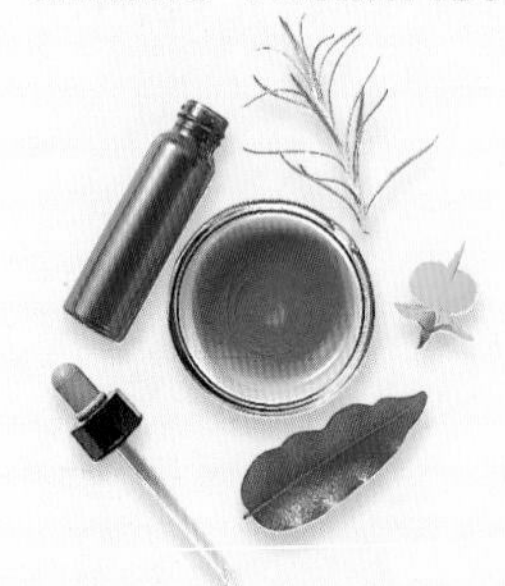

- Because homeopathy is a complete system of medicine in its own right, there is no point in mixing it with other systems such as acupuncture or herbalism. If you are using a number of different therapies, it's difficult to work out which one is really helping. Stick with the one that's helping! If it's not, move on.

DISCOVERING YOUR INDIVIDUAL RESPONSE THROUGH SYMPTOMS

We all respond in different ways, even if we are struggling with the same infection. Our unique responses form a pattern that corresponds to a picture of a homeopathic remedy. To find this pattern, you need to observe your preferences when ill – for example, what you want to drink, at what temperature you feel most comfortable, and whether you need fresh air. Some of us feel hot and feverish, while others become chilly and anxious. Most of us don't like to use up much-needed energy digesting food; some don't even want to drink. We may feel oversensitive to cold, but our nose might be less blocked in the open air. The art of using homeopathic remedies successfully depends on the ability to recognize the sometimes subtle ways we change when coping with illness.

HYPERICUM
ST JOHN'S WORT

QUESTIONS TO ASK IN THE CASE OF ACUTE INFECTIONS

- What triggered or caused this illness?
- What are the main symptoms bothering me?
- What are the other symptoms that have come on at the same time?
- If I have a pain – what sort of pain is it (e.g., sharp, dull, burning) and where is it located?
- If I have a cough – what sort of cough it is? (e.g., dry, mucous, painful)
- If I have a mucous discharge – what sort is it (color, odor, and whether it is irritating)?
- Is there any change in my body temperature; hotter, colder, or feverish?
- Is there any change in my physical appearance (pallor, redness, swelling, etc.)?
- At what time (day or night) do I feel worse?
- What makes me, or my symptoms, feel better?
- What makes me, or my symptoms, feel worse? (Consider position, movement, and temperature.)
- Has my mood changed – either before or since I started feeling ill?
- Is my appetite or thirst affected?
- Are my bowels affected? (Toward constipation or diarrhea?)

LEFT *The poison arsenic makes the valuable homeopathic remedy Arsenicum album. All remedies are completely safe to use in homeopathic dilutions.*

DOSAGE

- Take one tablet of the 6 potency three or four times daily for mild infections or to promote healing over a number of days. This would include such conditions as styes, colds, and knitting broken bones.
- Take one tablet of the 30 potency every two or three hours if in great discomfort. This includes situations such as painful injuries, high fevers, or severe food poisoning. Reduce the frequency as soon as you start feeling better.
- Be flexible regarding how often to take the remedy. Generally the worse the condition, the more frequently you need to take it – sometimes every hour or two until you see a response. In less urgent problems, take a 6 potency three times a day until improvement sets in, and then quickly tail off the remedy.
- Don't forget – the minimum dose that can achieve a cure is always the best.

Your emotional state provides important clues to choosing the right remedy for you. Homeopaths remember symptom pictures for each remedy as people. Do you get emotional and weepy like Pulsatilla, or anxious like Arsenicum and Phosphorus, who both worry a lot about being ill and need lots of reassurance? Or can you not bear to be fussed over, like Bryonia and Nux vomica, who get grumpy and irritable?

ACONITE

BELOW *Taking note of your symptoms is the first step to finding out what remedy you need.*

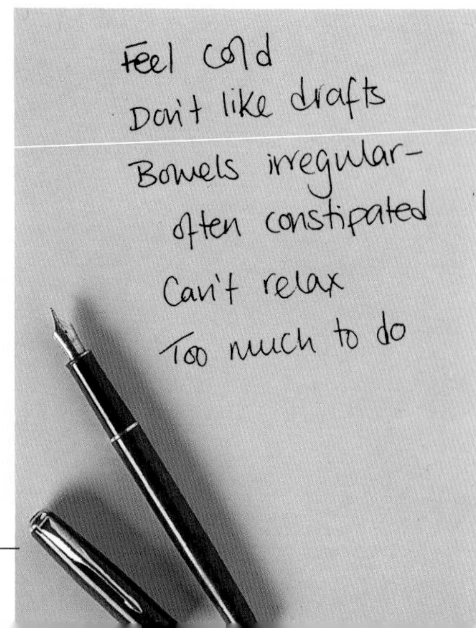

TAKING A REMEDY

- Remedies come in tablet form, or as granules for young children. Tinctures and creams are also available.

- The number printed on the label of any homeopathic medicine you buy indicates how many times it has been diluted and succussed. A 6 potency has been diluted six times, while a 30 has been diluted 30 times.

- One tablet (or a few granules) is enough for one dose. Dissolve the tablet under your tongue – without water. Crush it in paper for small children or babies, and try to avoid touching it with your own hands.

- Children can have a tablet dissolved in a small quantity of water but, again, don't touch the remedy with your own hands.

- Don't eat, drink, clean your teeth, or smoke for at least 20 minutes before or afterward, in case any strong substances in your mouth spoil the effectiveness of the remedy.

- Store the remedies in their original containers away from direct light, heat, and strong-smelling substances.

- In case of accidentally taking a number of remedies – don't panic. Taking dozens of tablets is no different to taking just one.

HOW TO TELL IF A REMEDY IS WORKING

When the remedy is working

- You feel better in yourself; your mood and energy are improving.
- The more unpleasant symptoms start clearing up first. For instance, if you have a fever, this subsides, although you may initially have more nasal discharge.
- Symptoms lessen in intensity.

When the remedy is not working

- You feel worse in yourself
- No change in the symptoms
- Symptoms get worse

Conclusion: The remedy has had no effect; try another one.

BELOW *Remedies are available as tablets, granules, tinctures, and creams.*

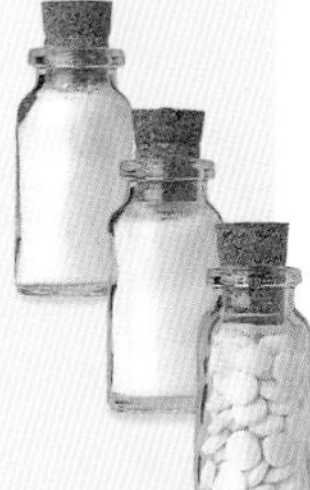

LEFT *Taking a remedy is easy. You don't need water – just dissolve it under your tongue.*

Materia medica

HOMEOPATHIC REMEDY *pictures give you information on the many different kinds of ailments a remedy can treat, as well as describing in detail the specific symptoms involved. These also include subjective symptoms. How you feel is considered an important aspect of illness, and tiredness or emotional changes often precede physical illness as early-warning signs. The following pages include some of the most commonly prescribed remedies, selected to cover physical and mental disorders that occur in a range of conditions.*

NUX VOMICA

PULSATILLA

PULSATILLA

- Gentle, sympathetic character
- Feels vulnerable and weepy
- Ailments are the result of feeling upset and emotional
- Feels much better in company
- Menstrual problems
- Warm-blooded – doesn't feel the cold
- Rich fatty foods aggravate the digestion
- Prefers bland food
- Symptoms better in cool, fresh air

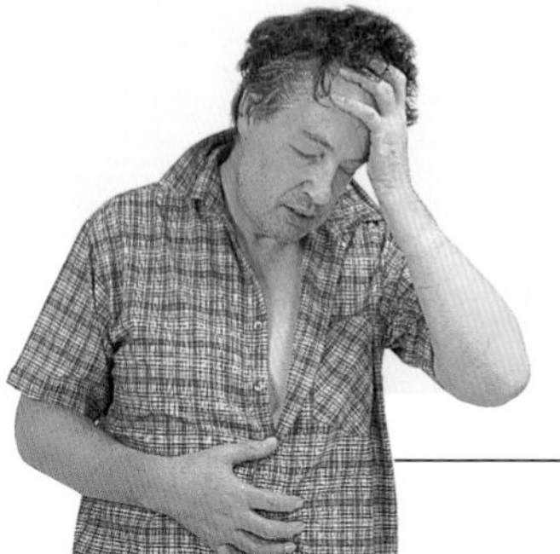

NUX VOMICA

- Oversensitive and impatient temperament
- Feels irritable and angry inside – even if not expressed
- Ailments are caused from stress
- Insomnia
- Gastric problems; indigestion, heartburn, ulcers, irritable bowel syndrome
- Constipation
- Chilly
- Likes fatty or spicy food, coffee, and alcohol
- Likes fresh air

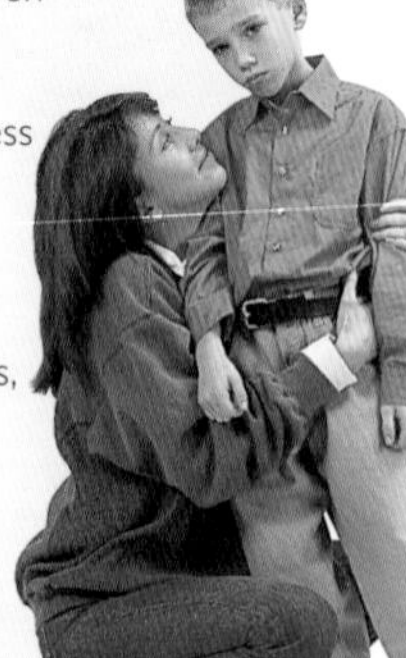

MATCHING REMEDY PICTURES

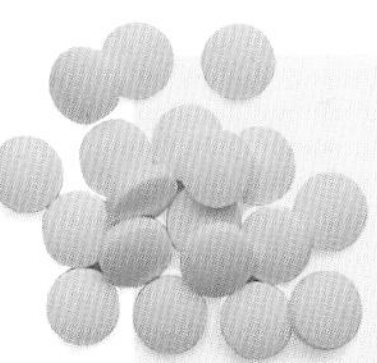

Belladonna in tablet form

You take the remedy that most closely matches your symptoms. Use the materia medica on pages 22–51 to identify the remedy you need by first reading through the pictures to familiarize yourself with the remedy profile. Match the subjective and physical symptoms to your own situation. Examples are given in the right-hand column.

- Your child is clingy and whiny, but doesn't complain of any specific pain. Pale and droopy. Doesn't want to be left alone. Not very thirsty. If you look at the remedy picture of Pulsatilla *(see page 46)*, you'll see that this is the right remedy for this situation.

- You are pale and tired, with frequent diarrhea. Your mouth feels dry but you only want to drink a few sips of water at a time. You feel anxious, and the creases in the sheet bother you. This situation would respond to Arsenicum *(see page 28)*.

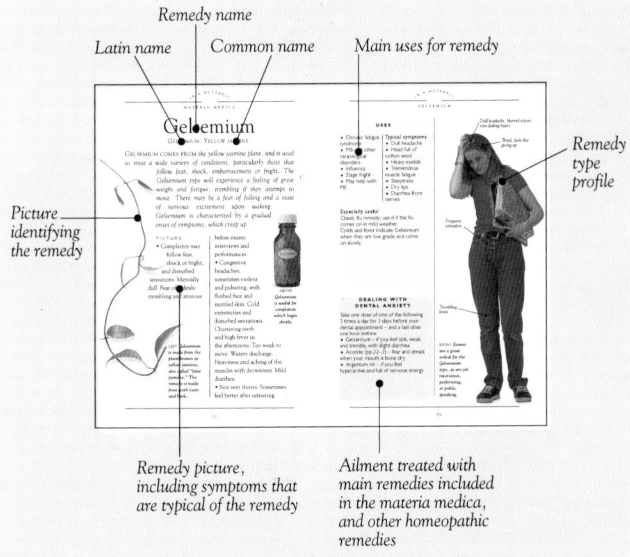

Aconite

ACONITUM NAPELLUS. MONKSHOOD.

ACONITE IS WIDELY *used by professional homeopaths for dramatic symptoms and conditions which arrive suddenly, with great intensity. The Aconite type is never feeble. Aconite would be prescribed constitutionally for someone healthy, rugged, robust and energetic, who is suffering from fears that have caused agitation.*

ABOVE ***The remedy is made from the flowering plant known as blue monkshood, so named because the poisonous flowers are shaped like a monk's hood. Aconite grows in mountainous places and it can help in shock following a fall.***

USES

- Panic attacks
- Shock
- Fevers

Beginning of infections, such as

- Sore throats
- Earaches
- Coughs and colds

QUICK REMEDY SPOTTER FOR COLDS

- Cold with fever: consider Aconite or Ferrum phos
- With streaming nose: compare Allium, Arsenicum (*pp.28–29*), Nux vomica (*pp.42–3*), Natrum mur, Euphrasia *(see Hay fever, page 55)*
- Thick catarrh: Dulcamara, Ant tart, Pulsatilla (*pp.46–7*), and Kali bich *(see Sinusitis, page 57)*.
- With conjunctivitis: Pulsatilla (*pp.46–7*)
- With cold sores: Natrum mur
- With nosebleeds: Ferrum phos, Phosphorus

PICTURE

• Psychological state is pronounced: fear they might die; panic attacks in elevators, subways, and planes; usually very anxious and restless, even with physical ailments; symptoms appear suddenly, often triggered by a fright, or by exposure to cold winds (such as Bell's palsy); panic attacks that come on after what feels like a near-death experience – such as a car accident.

• Helps at the beginning of colds; clear, hot, nasal discharge comes on straight after being chilled; feel feverish, with heat, chills, and restlessness; high fever with burning skin; sweaty and thirsty; head hot; headachey and dizzy; can also have earache, or sore throat; slight cough, which sounds hard and dry, described as "barking"; breathing in cold air brings on the cough; bright red inflammations.

• Thirsty, but everything tastes bitter except water.

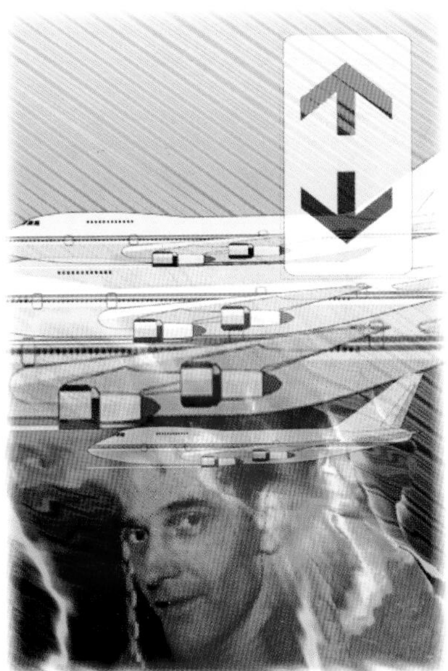

ABOVE ***Fearfulness is part of the Aconite remedy picture – especially feeling afraid of death after a shock.***

QUICK REMEDY SPOTTER FOR COUGHS

- Dry, tight: Aconite, Spongia, Hepar sulph
- Loose, wet, rattling cough: compare Ant tart and Pulsatilla (*pp.46–7*)
- Throaty: Rumex, Kali bich, Pulsatilla (*pp.46–7*)
- Chesty: Bryonia (*pp.32–3*) and Phosphorus (*pp.44–5*)

Apis

APIS MELLIFICA. HONEYBEE.

HOMEOPATHS USE APIS *mainly for allergic problems, as well as for cystitis and kidney infections. It may be needed following a fright, rage or in cases of jealousy (particularly sibling rivalry). The Apis mental state is characterized by restlessness and unpredictability. Apis would be appropriate for someone who craves company, but who rejects advances and affection. Fear of death is common in Apis types.*

ABOVE ***Apis is made from the honeybee, and its symptoms are similar to those caused by a bee sting.***

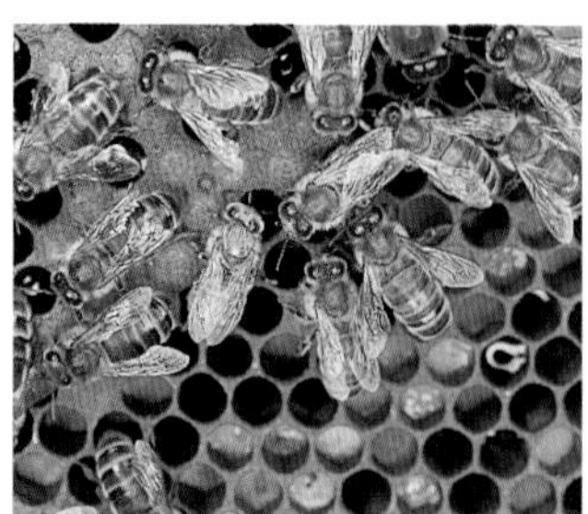

BELOW ***Apis is prepared from whole bees steeped in alcohol.***

Apis may be useful for ailments which involve watery swelling with edema (where the tissues are water-logged). The area will look red, shiny and puffy, with marked, rapid swelling. The remedy is made from the honeybee, so imagine a bee-sting and you'll be able to visualize the skin reactions that are likely to respond to this remedy. Apis can be used instead of antihistamines to relieve allergic skin reactions.

ALLERGIC SKIN REACTIONS

- Apis is used for allergic reactions to insect bites, where the skin swells up dramatically with a bright red, puffy appearance.
- For severe allergic reactions (anaphylaxis), which can lead to shock, give Apis 30 every 20 minutes and summon help.
- Urtica urens helps prickly heat during the summer, or "nettle rash" (hives) after eating foods like shellfish or strawberries.

PICTURE

• The mental picture is characterized by fidgeting and restlessness. There may be inappropriate emotional outbursts; moody. Jealousy, anger and tearfulness are symptoms.

• Physically, there will be pain that stings and burns. Symptoms will be better for cold; face flushed red, and rashes will be rough; tightness in the abdomen and scanty urine. Skin is sensitive to the touch, and hot and dry, or perspiring. Can be a little feverish and drowsy. Nausea, vomiting or retching, with great anxiety.

• There will be thirstlessness, and twitching in fever.

USES

- Bad reactions to insect bites or stings.
- Allergic skin rashes
- Mumps and measles

BELOW *Bee stings result in a hot, swollen skin reaction, especially if you have allergic tendencies.*

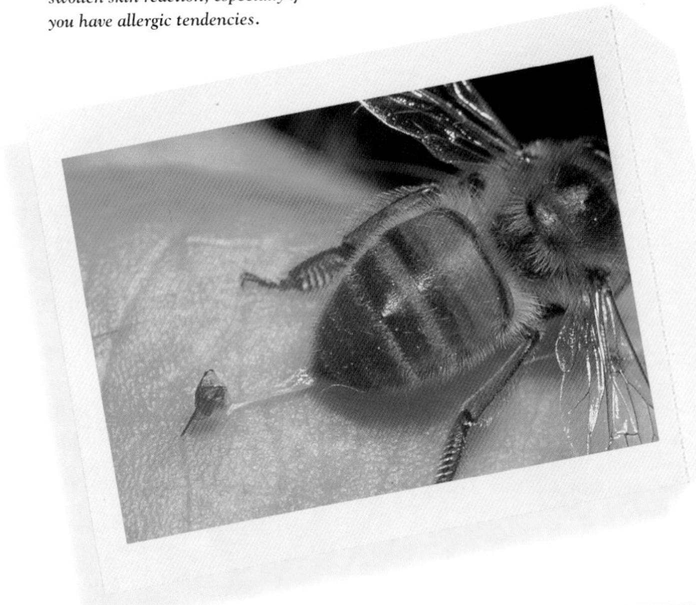

Arnica

ARNICA MONTANA. LEOPARDSBANE, OR "FALL" HERB.

ARNICA DESERVES ITS *reputation as the number-one remedy for accidents or injuries, along with the appropriate first aid treatment. It is useful for every kind of wound or injury, and helps recovery from physical and mental shock. The Arnica personality wants to be left alone, and fears contact because of pain or discomfort. Characteristically, Arnica is called for when the sufferer is averse to being talked to.*

PICTURE

- People needing Arnica typically have a stoical response to injuries; these are the people who get up after being knocked off their bicycles, saying, "I'm all right. There's really nothing wrong;" but some hours later the panic and shakiness start coming out; after an accident, a dose of Arnica 30 can be given every half hour on the way to hospital.

RIGHT ***Arnica is a member of the daisy family. It grows in mountainous regions and is sometimes called "fall" herb. It is very good for treating soft tissue damage after falls and accidents.***

SHOCK

- Arnica – after physical injuries. Helps bruising and soft tissue damage as well as shock
- Aconite (*pp.22–3*) – after a fright, where you feel overwhelmed by waves of anxiety and panic, with the feeling that you might have died
- Stramonium – after situations of pure terror, such as an attack or rape; nightmares, and can't sleep without the light on
- Ignatia – after bereavement; this is for grief or loss rather than fright; the person sighs a lot
- Staphysagria – after surgery, where you feel violated rather than shocked

The whole plant is used to make the remedy

The plant was often used as an infusion by South American Indians

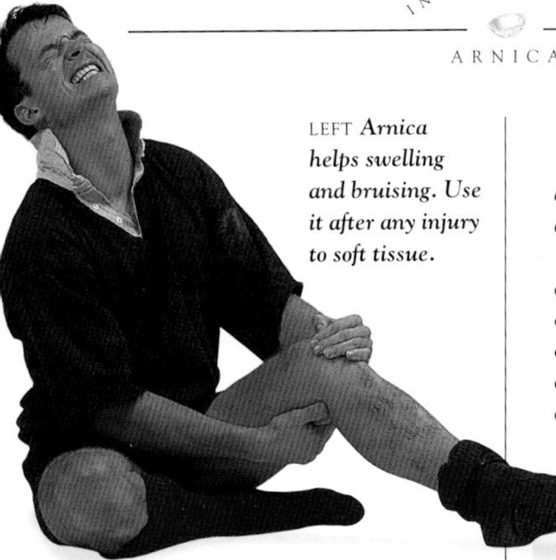

LEFT *Arnica helps swelling and bruising. Use it after any injury to soft tissue.*

•Mentally, Arnica patients will be weak, weary and seem stuporous, although able to answer questions.

• Physically, Arnica will be called for if there is a hot and red face and head, with cold extremities. There will be thirst and a feeling of chilliness. Joints may be swollen and sore; smelly discharges. The overwhelming feature which points to Arnica is great soreness and difficulty moving.

• Take Arnica for any damage to the soft tissues, because it helps with swelling and bruising. Useful after falls, blows, surgery, childbirth, dental extraction and other dental work, muscular strain or bruises of any nature.

USES

- Shock.
- Bruises, and other injuries where the skin isn't broken.
- Sprains with bruising.
- Arthritis with bruised feeling.
- After surgery.
- Aching with flu.
- After childbirth.

ACCIDENTS

• Arnica is used for blows to soft parts, with bruising and bleeding.

• Calendula is indicated for grazes and open wounds.

• Hypericum is for cuts to areas rich in nerves, or damage to the spine.

• Clean the area with Calendula lotion – a lotion is made from one part of the mother tincture to ten parts of water. In the case of cuts or puncture wounds you can moisten the dressing with Calendula lotion for the first day or two.

• After accidents Arnica can be taken in high potency for a few days, then another remedy can be taken in a low potency two or three times daily until better. For instance, in the case of a broken bone, take Arnica 30 three or four times daily until the swelling goes down, then switch to Symphytum 6 (made from comfrey or "bone-knit") for a few weeks to help bones knit together.

• In the case of a sprain, take Arnica 30 two or three times daily for a day or two, then Rhus tox 6 (*pp.48–9*) three times daily until the joint is mobile again.

Arsenicum

ARSENICUM ALBUM. ARSENIC TRIOXIDE.

ARSENICUM ALBUM IS USED *by homeopaths for many serious mental and emotional conditions, and matches the symptom picture characterized by anxiety, restlessness, burning pains which are better for heat, and weakness out of proportion to the illness. The Arsenicum type is fussy and perfectionist, fearing night, being alone and fate.*

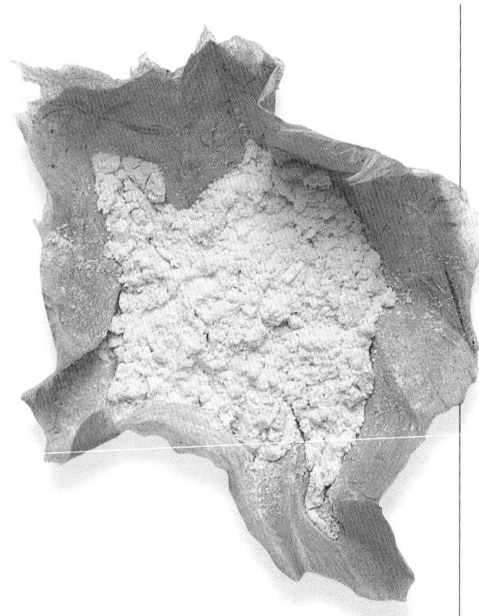

ABOVE **Arsenicum is made from the trioxide of arsenic, a poisonous substance that was proved by Hahnemann himself.**

PICTURE

- Generally weak and tired, but restless because of their anxious mental state; these are the types who must straighten out the room before they can take to their bed when ill. They are anxious about illness, or when ill; anxious about recovering (even from a minor ailment) and need a lot of reassurance.

USES

- Anxiety
- Food poisoning and diarrhea
- Hay fever
- Asthma
- Colds: typical Arsenicum cold is a head cold with watery discharge from the nose – which burns the upper lip
- Hay fever; lot of sneezing; the nose feels very hot and irritated inside

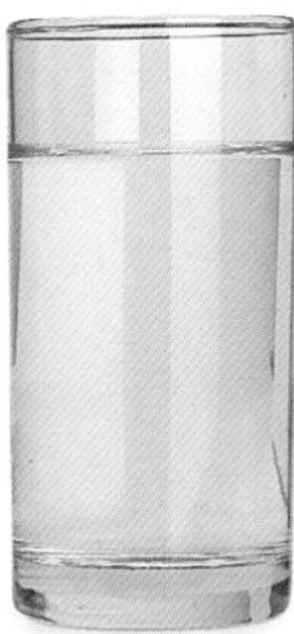

ABOVE ***The mouth feels dry but when Arsenicum is indicated, the patient only likes to sip small amounts of water.***

• Physical symptoms include chills with a sensation of ice water running in the veins and then an intense, high fever. Burning pains better for heat; discharges are acid and burning. Coughs are dry and hacking, with burning in the chest, difficulty breathing, wheezing. Vomiting everything with dry mouth, burning pains, gastritis, diarrhea which is worse for eating or drinking.

• Worse for cold air, better for warm. Skin often pale and clammy. Restless, thirsts for sips of ice-cold water.

FOOD POISONING

• Arsenicum – diarrhea with vomiting, prostration, or anxiety. Any stools are painless, scanty, brown, and smelly, and may burn the anus

• Veratrum – diarrhea and vomiting at the same time. Abdominal cramps and cold shivers

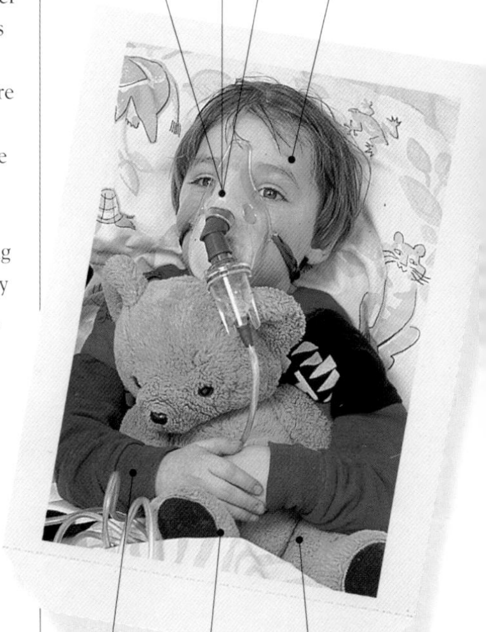

Right side of nose may be blocked up

Sneezing

Hot discharge from nose

Head feels better for cold air

Anxious and restless

Chilly and likes to be warm

Feels run down

ABOVE **An Arsenicum-type head cold is characterized by a watery discharge which burns.**

Belladonna

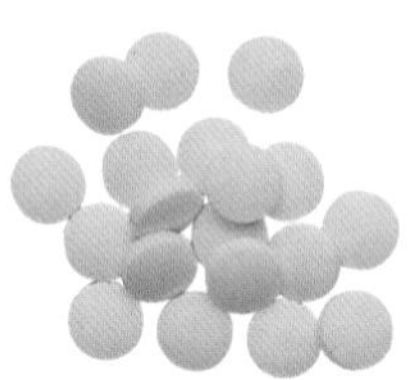

ABOVE **In homeopathic form, Belladonna is safe and effective – indeed it is commonly prescribed for children.**

BELLADONNA. DEADLY NIGHTSHADE.

BELLADONNA, WHICH IS *produced from the deadly nightshade plant, is suitable for conditions which come on suddenly and vehemently, and then subside as quickly. The constitutional type is similar to Aconite, in that it is suited to healthy, vigorous people. When well the Belladonna type is charming, friendly and cheerful; when unwell, these people are violent and moody.*

PICTURE

- Mental picture includes a great sensitivity to pains, which come and go quickly. Violence and occasionally delirium. Hypersensitivity to noise and to bright light.
- Symptoms are intense, coming on rapidly; a high fever develops, with burning skin; the head is often very hot, radiating heat, while the feet and hands are cool to touch; look hot

USES

- Fever, with a high temperature. Infections and childhood illnesses that come on suddenly, with a fever
- Migraines, with sensitivity to noise, touch and light

Belladonna, made from the poisonous deadly nightshade plant

RIGHT **In homeopathic form, even medicines made from poisonous substances are completely nontoxic.**

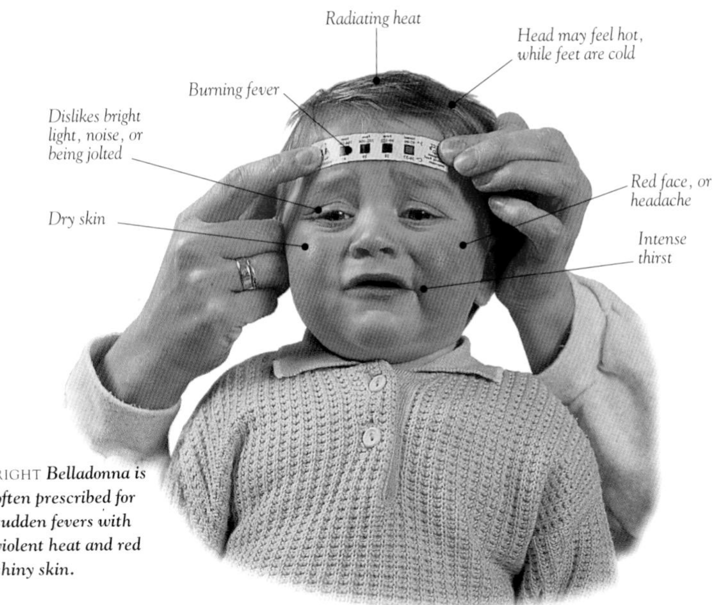

RIGHT **Belladonna is often prescribed for sudden fevers with violent heat and red shiny skin.**

and flushed, with dry skin; glassy eyes with dilated pupils; may complain of a throbbing headache; breathing may be shallow and rapid; throat feels hot and painful; it's difficult to swallow; dry; despite their heat, there is no sweating, and often no thirst – or thirst for lots of cold water or lemonade.

- Worse for motion, and worse at 3 pm and at night. Very sensitive to touch.

MASTITIS

- Belladonna – with high temperature
- Bryonia (*pp.32-3*) – feverish; breasts so painful can't feed or express milk
- Phytolacca – breasts and glands in armpit and sometimes neck feels very swollen and tender; feels fluish
- Phytolacca can also be taken in tincture form, 5 drops three times a day

Bryonia

BRYONIA ALBA. WHITE BRYONY.

BRYONIA WAS ONE *of the first homeopathic remedies proved by Hahnemann, and has been widely used for many conditions over the past 100 years. The main symptom picture is complaints that begin a day or so after exposure to cold, or to dry, cold winds. Complaints come on slowly, and may be chronic. Complaints often begin in the morning, and cause the sufferer to feel tired, slow, and unable to think clearly.*

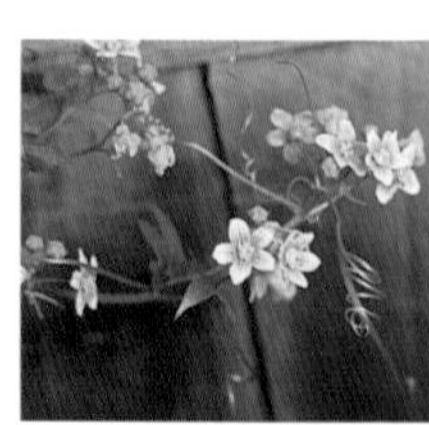

ABOVE **The flowers of white bryony blossom in early summer**

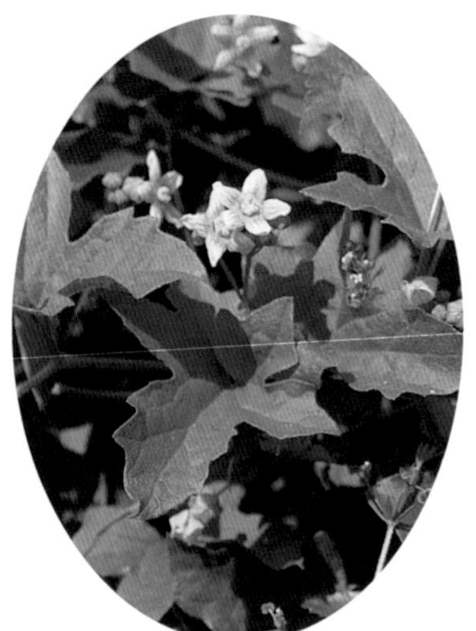

ABOVE **Bryonia is made from the white bryony, a climbing plant found throughout Europe.**

PICTURE

- Irritable, and hate to be fussed over; continue to worry about work even when too ill to do anything about it; worry about money.
- Affected parts of the body feel dry, whether nose, throat, respiratory tract or joints; can get constipated, with hard dry stools

USES

- Dry cough
- Headaches and constipation
- Arthritis
- Pleurisy, bronchitis, asthma, and whooping cough
- Lung, digestive and arthritic complaints

that look like sheep's droppings; thirsty; want plenty of cold water; lips dry; flu which comes on gradually, making them increasingly irritable; the cough is dry, and hurts the chest (or head) so that they hold the chest when coughing; moving around, or coming into a warm room brings on the cough; experienced homeopaths can use this remedy to treat pleurisy and pneumonia characterized by a stitching pain felt with every breath; bad headache, worse with every movement – even of the eyes.

• Worse for motion, heat and stuffy rooms. Better for pressure. Great thirst for lots of cold water.

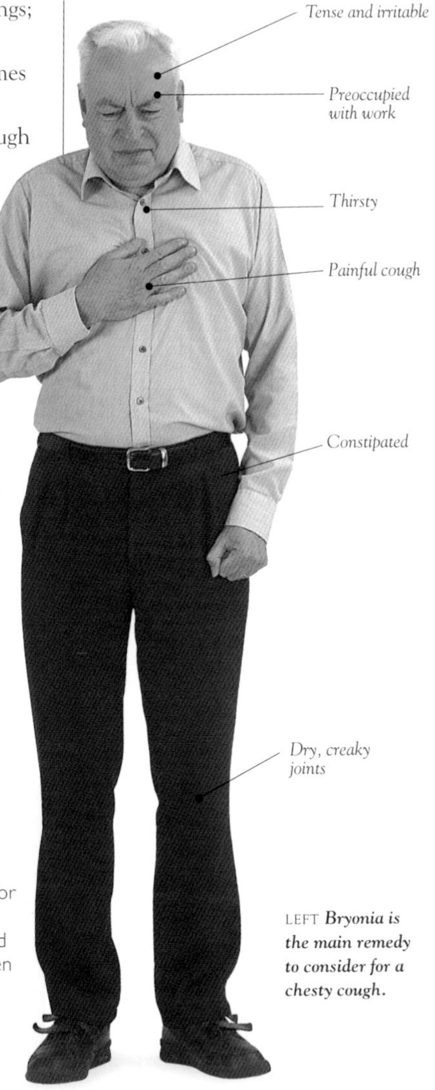

LEFT ***Bryonia is the main remedy to consider for a chesty cough.***

CONSTIPATION

- Bryonia – for hard stools like sheep's droppings
- Nux vomica (*pp.42–3*) – for when you can't move bowels even though you feel the need
- Silica (*pp.50–51*) – for when you try to move bowels, but stool seems to slip back in

Calendula

CALENDULA OFFICINALIS. MARIGOLD.

CALENDULA IS THE *mainstay of any good homeopathic first aid kit, and can be used on all minor cuts, grazes, shallow wounds, and scalds. Because it is primarily a first aid remedy, there is no real psychological picture. The remedy is suitable for anyone suffering from minor wounds.*

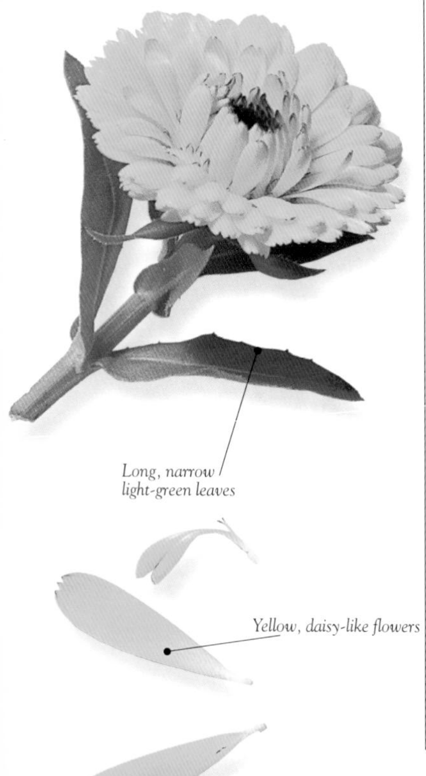

PICTURE

- Excessive pain, which is out of proportion to the injury.
- The antiseptic properties of Calendula prevent wounds from getting infected; it aids healing, and encourages the formation of healthy scar tissue; apply a lotion made from diluted tincture (one part tincture to ten parts water) to grazed skin; this lotion can also be used as a mouthwash after dental work has been done, either on its own, or mixed with the same amount of Hypericum; Calendula talc (in a talcum powder base) is effective

LEFT ***Calendula is made from the leaves and flowers of the common marigold plant.***

in relieving athlete's foot; sprinkle some talc between the toes after every bath or shower – or before any exertion that will make your feet sweat; Calendula is also useful after childbirth and tooth extraction where there is much bleeding.

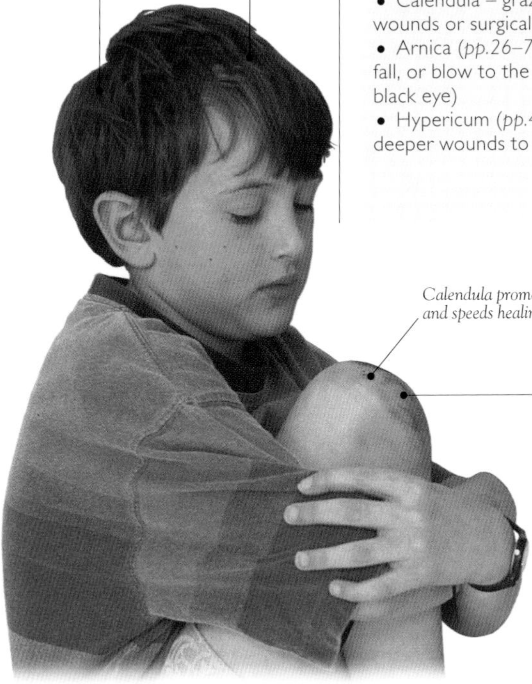

USES

- Injuries, where the skin is broken.
- Grazes and sores
- Any type of cut or sore where the skin is broken. It should be compared with Hypericum

WOUNDS

- Remedies can be taken along with appropriate first aid measures
- Calendula – grazes; or when wounds or surgical scars look inflamed
- Arnica (*pp.26–7*) – take it after any fall, or blow to the body (including a black eye)
- Hypericum (*pp.40–41*) – cuts and deeper wounds to parts rich in nerves

May be irritable or frightened

Excessive pain – out of proportion to injury

Calendula promotes and speeds healing

Helps clot formation and keeps wounds clean

LEFT ***Calendula is a good antiseptic, and helps grazed skin to heal cleanly.***

Chamomilla

CHAMOMILLA. CHAMOMILE.

CHAMOMILLA, *from the wild chamomile plant, is an important remedy for nervous disorders, and for many childhood complaints such as colic, teething, and earache. Chamomilla is indicated when the sufferer is enormously sensitive, irritable, and has a low pain threshold. It can also be used for behavioral problems in children, PMS in women, and digestive disorders in people of every age.*

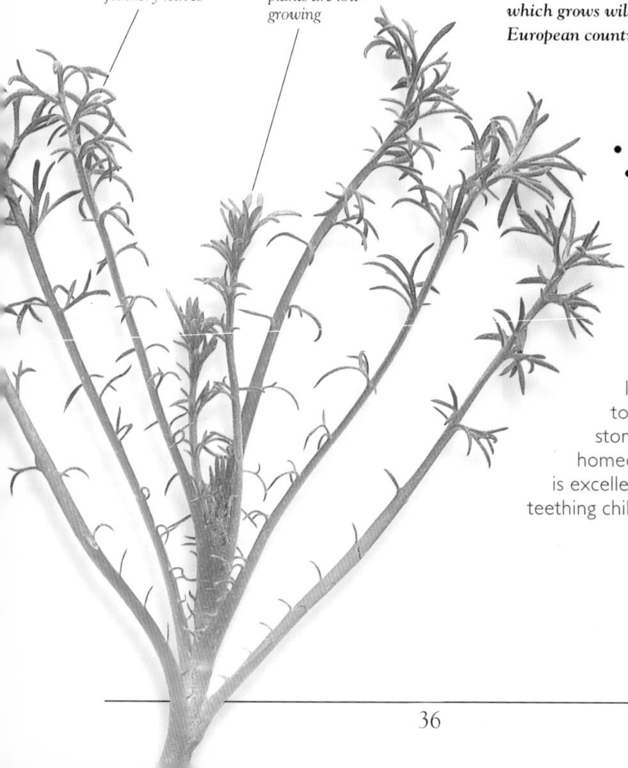

The plant has feathery leaves

Chamomile plants are low-growing

LEFT ***Chamomilla is another member of the daisy family, which grows wild in European countries.***

USES

- Diarrhea
- Toothache
- Colic
- Earache
- Nervous or psychological afflictions

Chamomile infusions have long been drunk to calm upset stomachs, and in homeopathic form it is excellent for soothing teething children.

PICTURE

• Child-type is irritable, demanding, and inconsolable, wants to be carried, low pain threshold; useful for teething, diarrhea with greenish stools; especially useful for infant teething, or colic accompanied by rotten-smelling stools that look like chopped spinach; "teething granules" are made in a form that's easy for infants to take; perhaps it's the low pain threshold that makes the Chamomilla-type complain so much; they feel very irritable and bad-tempered, just looking at, or speaking to the child is enough to send them off into a temper tantrum, it's hard to placate them because they don't know what they want; pushing away anything you offer; the only thing that settles them is being carried about or rocked.

• Either restless, or drowsy, moaning in sleep; flushed, red face; one cheek red and hot, the other pale; feel worse when they get too hot.

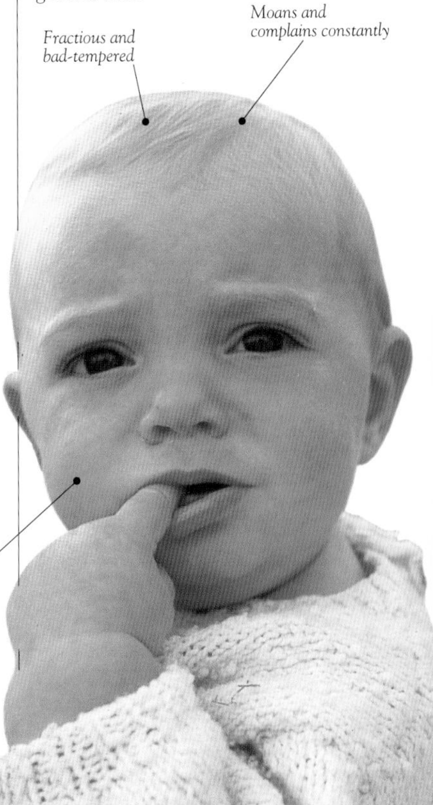

RIGHT ***Chamomilla teething granules are excellent for soothing a teething child and ease the discomfort. They also help other symptoms that come on with teething, including mild fever, skin rashes, and diarrhea.***

Gelsemium

GELSEMIUM. YELLOW JASMINE.

GELSEMIUM COMES FROM *the yellow jasmine plant, and is used to treat a wide variety of conditions, particularly those that follow fear, shock, embarrassment or fright. The Gelsemium type will experience a feeling of great weight and fatigue, trembling if they attempt to move. There may be a fear of falling and a state of nervous excitement upon waking. Gelsemium is characterized by a gradual onset of symptoms, which creep up.*

PICTURE

• Complaints may follow fear, shock or fright, and disturbed sensations. Mentally dull. Fear of ordeals: trembling and anxious before exams, interviews and performances.

• Congestive headaches, sometimes violent and pulsating, with flushed face and mottled skin. Cold extremities and disturbed sensations. Chattering teeth and high fever in the afternoons. Too weak to move. Watery discharge. Heaviness and aching of the muscles with drowsiness. Mild diarrhea.

• Not very thirsty. Sometimes feel better after urinating.

LEFT ***Gelsemium is made from the plant known as yellow jasmine, also called "false jasmine." The remedy is made from fresh roots and bark.***

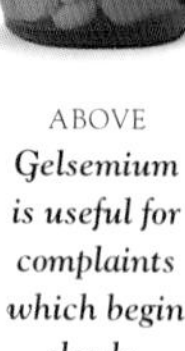

ABOVE ***Gelsemium is useful for complaints which begin slowly.***

USES

- Chronic fatigue syndrome
- MS and other neurological disorders
- Influenza
- Stage fright
- May help with ME

Typical symptoms
- Dull headache
- Head feels full of cotton wool
- Heavy eyelids
- Tremendous muscle fatigue
- Sleepiness
- Dry lips
- Diarrhea from nerves

Especially useful
Classic flu remedy; use it if the flu comes on in mild weather.
Colds and fever indicate Gelsemium when they are low grade and come on slowly.

DEALING WITH DENTAL ANXIETY

Take one dose of one of the following 3 times a day for 3 days before your dental appointment – and a last dose one hour before:
- Gelsemium – if you feel sick, weak, and trembly, with slight diarrhea
- Aconite (*pp.22–3*) – fear and dread, when your mouth is bone dry
- Argentum nit – if you feel hyperactive and full of nervous energy

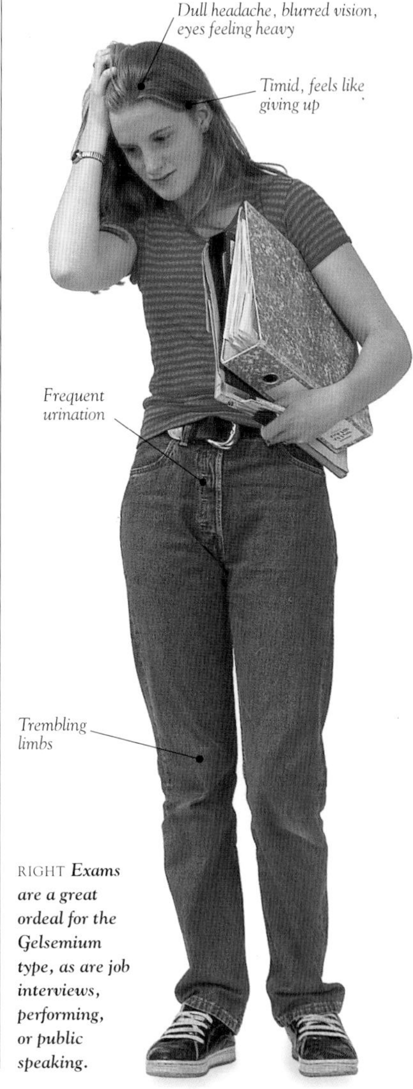

RIGHT ***Exams are a great ordeal for the Gelsemium type, as are job interviews, performing, or public speaking.***

Hypericum

HYPERICUM. SAINT-JOHN'S-WORT.

HYPERICUM IS USED *mainly as a first aid remedy, particularly when there is damage to the head, spine or coccyx, or parts of the body with many nerves, such as the lips, fingers and toes. The key symptoms that indicate Hypericum are excessive nerve pains that shoot upwards. Because Hypericum is mainly a first aid remedy, there is no clear-cut mental picture, although severe depression or impaired memory following injury may occur.*

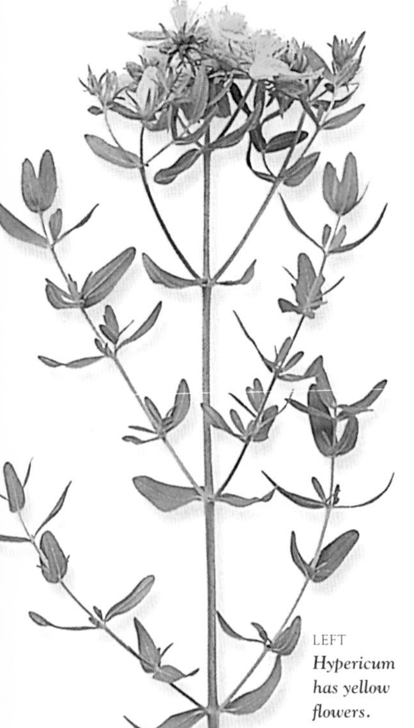

LEFT ***Hypericum has yellow flowers.***

PICTURE

- Nerve pains, where the pain seems to shoot along the nerve paths; it's for puncture wounds – so take a dose any time you step on a sharp object; it has a reputation as a remedy against tetanus; pain in the coccyx after a fall, or after childbirth; after dental work, use a mouthwash of Hypericum and Calendula mixed – known as Hyperical (one part of tincture is mixed with 10 parts of water); this is antibacterial, antiviral, and also anesthetizes any sensitive areas in the mouth.
- Pain worse for motion and pressure. Better for keeping still and lying on the painful side.

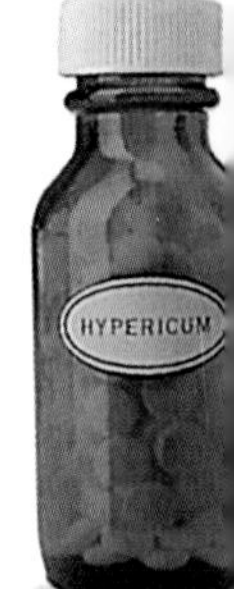

ABOVE ***Hyperic[um] is made from t[he] whole, fresh pl[ant] of Saint-John's-wort.***

SAINT-JOHN'S-WORT

Saint-John's-wort is used to make the homeopathic remedy Hypericum, and is particularly good where tissues are badly damaged. As a herb Saint-John's-wort can be used in an infusion, tincture, or oil, and is often given when people need revitalizing. Saint-John's-wort is, among other things, a natural antidepressant and nerve tonic. It is also used on a poor, sluggish digestion, and for insomnia or poor memory.

USES

- Injuries, especially deep injuries in sensitive parts of the body
- Any injuries to fingertips, toes, lips, ears, and tailbone (coccyx)

INJURIES

Cuts
Hypericum – for cuts and deeper wounds to parts rich in nerves, such as from stepping on a sharp object

Grazes
Calendula (*pp.34–5*) – take it whenever wounds or surgical scars look inflamed and infected

Blows
Arnica (*pp.26–7*) – deals with mental shock, as well as swelling and bruising. It promotes the reabsorption of blood from the tissues. Take it after any fall, or blow to the body (including a black eye)

INDICATIONS

Symptoms are made worse from motion, fear, shock, touch, exertion, change of weather, cold, and damp

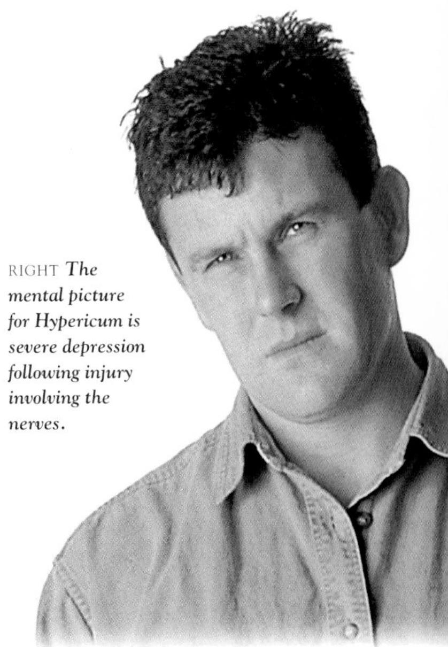

RIGHT ***The mental picture for Hypericum is severe depression following injury involving the nerves.***

Nux vomica

NUX VOMICA. POISON NUT TREE.

NUX VOMICA IS ONE *of the most important homeopathic remedies, and it is used for a wide variety of mental, emotional, and physical symptoms. It is perhaps the most appropriate remedy for people who work hard – burning the candle at both ends, and suffering from high levels of stress. The Nux vomica type is fussy, a workaholic, and given to outbursts of anger. These people are unable to take criticism, and take on too much.*

Nux vomica is made from the seeds of the poison nut tree

LEFT ***Nux vomica was first proved by Hahnemann himself, from the seeds of the poison nut tree which contain strychnine, a powerful poison which works on the central nervous system.***

USES

- Indigestion
- Nausea
- Hangover
- Tension
- Headaches
- Colds and flu
- Catarrh
- Coughs
- Head colds
- Insomnia
- Irritable bowel syndrome
- Backache

PICTURE

- Difficulty relaxing; insomnia; wake in the early hours (particularly around 3 am), often worrying about work; irritable and argumentative; best left alone when ill; often feel a lot of suppressed anger inside, which may erupt occasionally.
- Colds; blocked nose, which runs in a warm room; dry, tickly cough; throat dry and raw; nose streams like a tap; sneezing; chilly body, need to be warm; very sensitive to cold and drafts of air; usually constipated; feel blocked up; in irritable bowel syndrome the constipation may alternate with diarrhea; spasms and cramp in intestines, especially after too much rich food and stimulants; if this picture occurs before periods, Nux vomica can help PMS.
- Worse for cold.
- This remedy is usually needed when overindulgence in spicy food, coffee, or alcohol, or too much stress, lead to a hyped-up nervous system.

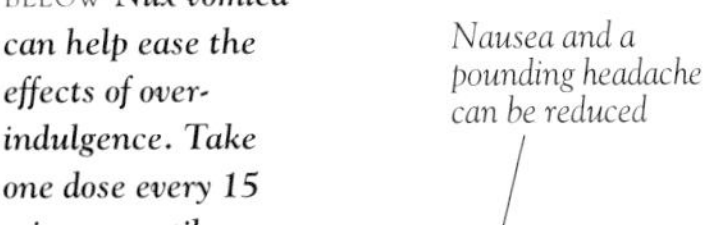

BELOW ***Nux vomica can help ease the effects of over-indulgence. Take one dose every 15 minutes until symptoms subside.***

INDIGESTION

- Nux vomica – food lies like a load in the stomach; want to vomit but can't; heartburn – aggravated by spirits, tobacco, coffee, rich or spicy foods
- Lycopodium – feel very full up after eating a small amount; lot of bloating and wind, especially after eating cabbage
- Bryonia (*pp.32–3*) – heaviness and queasiness; aggravated by vinegar or oysters.
- Pulsatilla (*pp.46–7*) – rich, fatty food causes indigestion

Phosphorus

PHOSPHORUS. PHOSPHORUS.

PHOSPHORUS IS A VERY *important homeopathic remedy, and is used for conditions ranging from sleep disorders, psoriasis and diabetes, to pneumonia. Even conditions as serious as manic depression or tuberculosis respond to this remedy. The Phosphorus type is normally intelligent and affectionate, but easily tired and liable to become moody.*

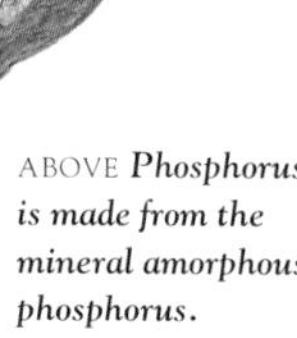

ABOVE ***Phosphorus is made from the mineral amorphous phosphorus.***

USES

- Nausea
- Vomiting
- Diarrhea
- Nosebleeds
- Period pains
- Headaches
- Dry skin
- Pneumonia
- Acute asthma
- Cramps
- Heartburn
- Sexual problems

The Phosphorus picture is one of extroversion: when healthy, the Phosphorus type is bubbly and outgoing. These people may be emotionally oversensitive to the problems of others, and sometimes even develop symptoms in sympathy. There is often a free-floating anxiety which easily attaches itself to minor physical symptoms; outbursts of rage, balanced by distress, and embarrassment. Phosphorus is excellent for nervous tension, particularly caused by overwork. It is also used to treat deep-seated fears, such as fear of the dark, or dying. It is a commonly used "constitutional" remedy.

PICTURE

- Sensitivity to external stimuli.
- Exhausted by a constant cough; tickly cough in delicate people with weak chests; hard, barking cough made worse by talking, laughing, in open air; cough can be triggered by any change in temperature – for instance, coming into a warm room from outdoors; very thirsty, especially for iced drinks; love ice and ice-cream when ill; distended blood vessels cause sudden nosebleeds, or traces of fresh blood in the phlegm.
- Chest feels constricted; suffocation better for pressure. Flushes of blood and heat going upwards. Violent palpitations.
- Hunger, violent thirst for ice-cold drinks. Hoarseness, worse in the evening. Complaints may come on from changes in the atmosphere.

NAUSEA AND VOMITING

- Phosphorus – severe nausea; vomits everything, even water
- Colocynth – vomiting from intense stomach cramps; have to double up

BELOW ***When healthy, Phosphorus people are active and lively. When ill, all their energy seems to drain away.***

Easily refreshed by sleep
Enthusiastic and sympathetic nature
Eats well but doesn't gain weight

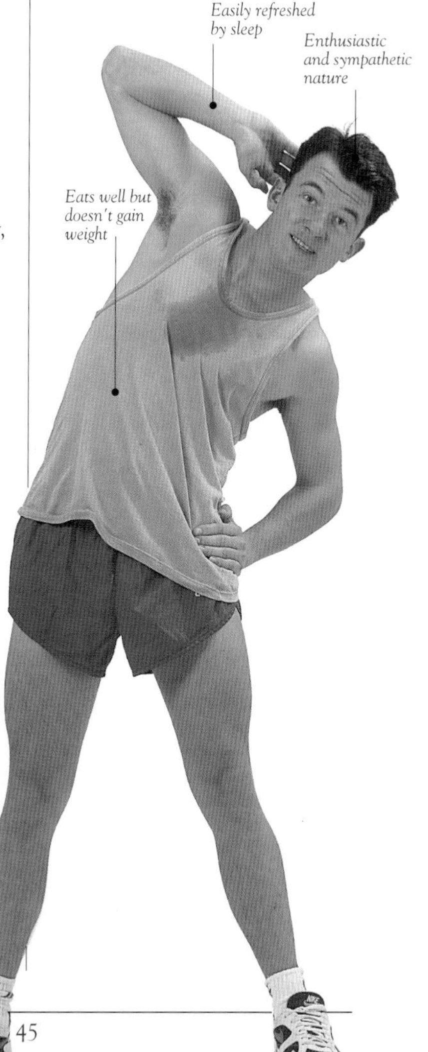

Pulsatilla

PULSATILLA. PASQUEFLOWER OR WINDFLOWER.

The remedy is prepared from the whole fresh plant
The finely cut leaves move in the wind

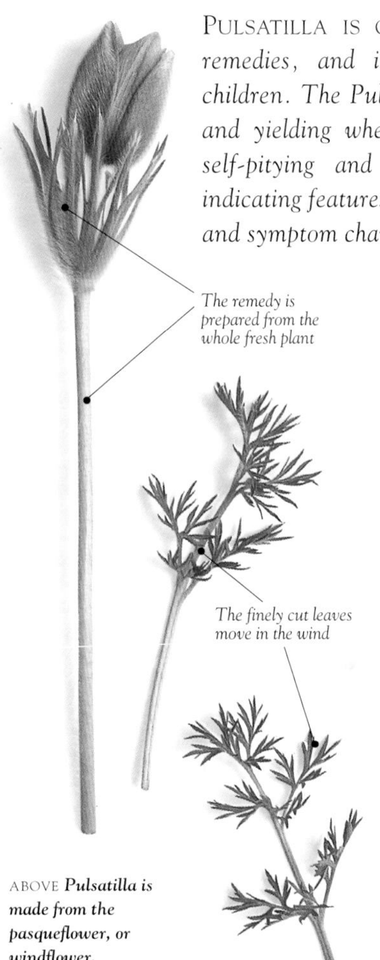

ABOVE ***Pulsatilla is made from the pasqueflower, or windflower.***

PULSATILLA IS ONE OF *the major homeopathic remedies, and is often used for women and children. The Pulsatilla personality is gentle, mild and yielding when well, and desiring attention, self-pitying and moody when ill. The main indicating features for this remedy are erratic mood and symptom changes.*

PICTURE

- The Pulsatilla emotional state is one of over-sensitivity and tears; when unwell like to be looked after and made a fuss of; children are mild and weepy, and want to be cuddled constantly.
- Helps in childhood illnesses where the child has mild fevers, a

USES OF PULSATILLA

- Weepy depression
- Menstrual problems
- Thrush and cystitis
- Gastric disorders
- Earaches
- Sleep disorders

Childhood illnesses, including:
- Measles
- Mumps
- Chicken pox
- Earaches
- Colds
- Conjunctivitis
- Styes

runny nose, and is very clingy and whiny; the face may appear hot and flushed; patient feels warm; worse in a warm room and wants the windows open; mucous: thick yellow catarrh hangs from nose or runny nose, with thick yellow or green mucus, and a cough which comes on lying down at night; the cold may affect the ears. This is the main remedy for a loose cough with lots of mucus – thick and often yellow-green; nose stuffed up in a warm room, and at night so it's difficult to sleep; nose runs in the open air; the child feels better walking in the open air; has little thirst, despite dry mouth.

- In conjunctivitis a little mucus accumulates in the corner of the eye; in thrush, thick creamy, or heavy yellowish discharge; helps bouts of thrush and cystitis, or PMS if a Pulsatilla-type mood comes on premenstrually.
- Better for slow, gentle motion; thirstlessness; worse for heat; desires cool, open air; one-sided complaints; worse for rich and fatty foods. Digestive complaints worse in the morning; mental complaints worse in the evening.

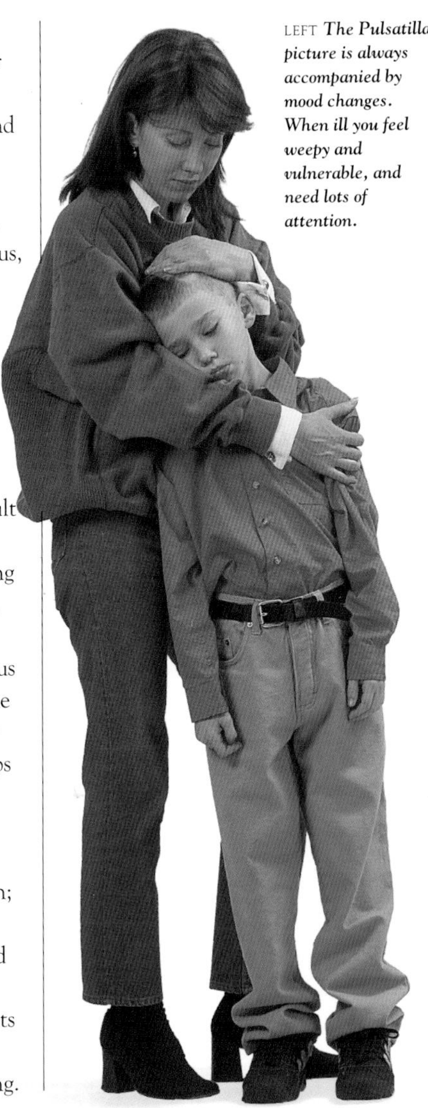

LEFT *The Pulsatilla picture is always accompanied by mood changes. When ill you feel weepy and vulnerable, and need lots of attention.*

Rhus tox

RHUS TOXICODENDRON. POISON IVY.

RHUS TOX IS SUITABLE *for any conditions afflicting the joints, ligaments, tendons and skin. The Rhus tox personality is restless, depressed, worried, and often overly suspicious.*

ABOVE ***Rhus tox is made from the leaves of the poison ivy and the poison oak plants, which are both natives of North America.***

BELOW ***Poison oak and poison ivy are closely related plants.***

PICTURE

- The mental picture is restless, anxious, aching, and with sore, tearing pains. A feeling of chilliness, and feeling of being stupefied. Sufferers spend time worrying about other people.
- Flu, feverish with aching limbs and bones; viral infections that involve the joints; runny nose and dry cough, especially when feeling cold; fever blisters or cold sores that erupt around the mouth.

USES

- Shingles and herpes
- Sprains and strains
- Flu
- Chicken pox
- Arthritis
- Urticaria
- Coughs

• Rheumatism and arthritis, where the joint pains are worse for lying in one position for too long, can be treated with Rhus tox. Small of the back very stiff; symptoms which begin after a sprain or injury.

• Useful for itchy, red rashes caused by allergies. Rash can appear over joints. Eruptions are red, itchy and often blistered; red, triangular tip to the tongue. Soothes itching and eruptions in chicken pox and shingles.

• Better for heat and motion, worse for cold. Thirsty, sometimes for milk. Joints are worse in damp, cold weather, and in the morning.

IMPETIGO

- Rhus tox – fever blisters around the lips or at the tip of the nose
- Ant tart – nasal discharge
- Arum triphyllum – red, irritated skin round mouth and chin, with cracked lips

SHINGLES

- Rhus tox – shingles with a lot of aching and restlessness; feels fluey
- Ranunculus – shingles with severe nerve pain
- Arsenicum (*pp.28–9*) – very painful; burning, and better from hot applications
- Apis (*pp.24–5*) – where the skin is very swollen and inflamed; blisters can ulcerate

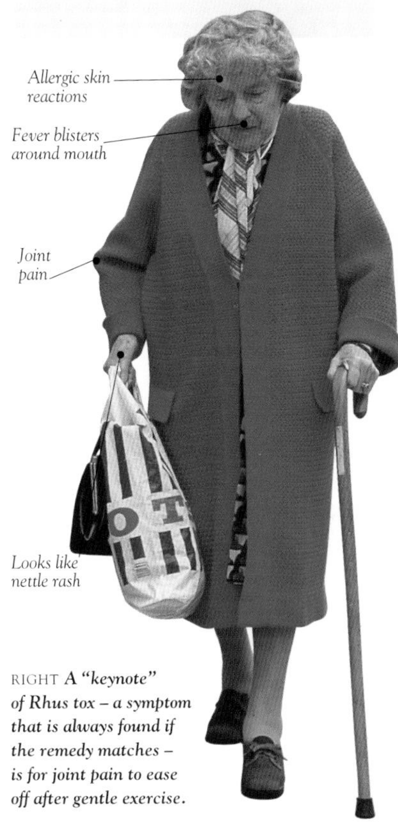

RIGHT ***A "keynote" of Rhus tox – a symptom that is always found if the remedy matches – is for joint pain to ease off after gentle exercise.***

Silica

SILICEA. FLINT.

SILICA IS A MAJOR *homeopathic remedy that is suited to complaints that develop slowly, and chronic conditions. It has an affinity with the digestive system, and is excellent for promoting the expulsion of foreign bodies, such as splinters. The Silica type is self-willed but lacking self-confidence, frightened to attempt new things, and continually tired; likes to sit and do nothing, but defensive about lack of drive.*

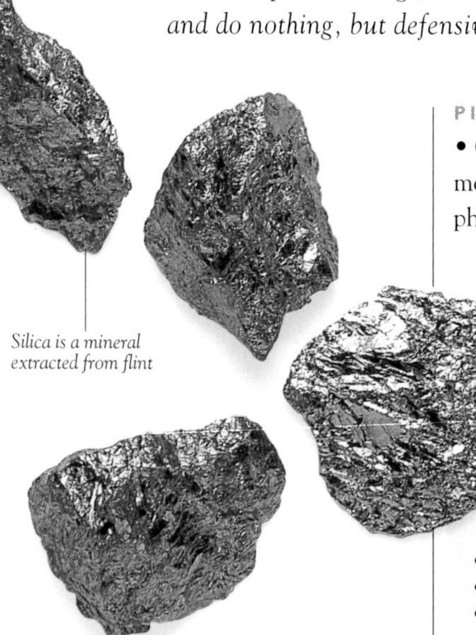

Silica is a mineral extracted from flint

ABOVE ***A substance that seems inert, like flint, can produce a remedy that stimulates healing when prepared homeopathically.***

PICTURE

- Children may be bright mentally, but fail to thrive physically. Stubborn, shy or timid. Lacking self-confidence. Weak and pale, with no stamina. Fear of needles.
- Wounds are slow to heal, or tend to get

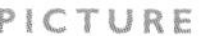

USES OF SILICA

- Colds that don't clear up
- Boils
- Dental abscesses
- Slow healing
- Headache
- Offensive sweat
- Chronic ear discharge
- Digestive disorders

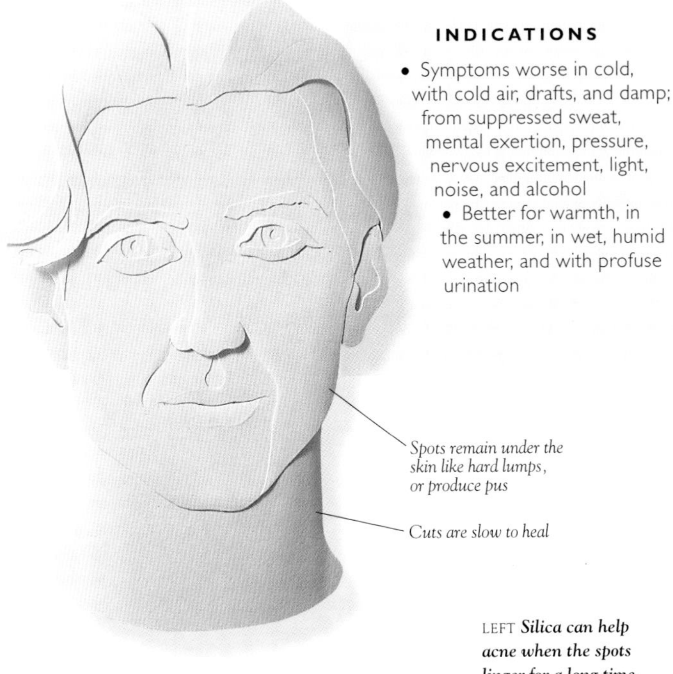

INDICATIONS

- Symptoms worse in cold, with cold air, drafts, and damp; from suppressed sweat, mental exertion, pressure, nervous excitement, light, noise, and alcohol
- Better for warmth, in the summer, in wet, humid weather, and with profuse urination

LEFT ***Silica can help acne when the spots linger for a long time.***

infected. Cuts don't seem to heal, scars look red and angry. Old scars reactivate. Splinters that are stuck under the skin can be pushed out with Silica. Abscesses that are slow to come to a head, or recurrent, or constantly becoming re-infected. Thick yellow discharge, enlarged lymph nodes, and offensive sweat about the upper part of the body or head. Headache from the back of the head, going over to the forehead. Lingering colds, dried mucus, eventually earache and chronic ear discharges; weak nails, which break easily.

- Symptoms often come on in cold, damp weather. Improved by cold, dry weather. Symptoms worse after getting feet wet, or suppressing sweat.

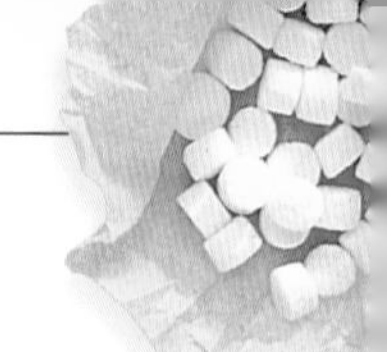

Home use

MILD INFECTIONS *and other minor ailments are safe to treat at home. This guide will give simple suggestions for common self-help remedies for some of the conditions that can be treated at home. If a remedy is described more fully in the materia medica section* (see pages 20–51)*, you can use the extra information to help make a decision about whether it's the right one for you.*

BELOW ***Your illness or health condition will dictate the potency and the form in which you take the remedies.***

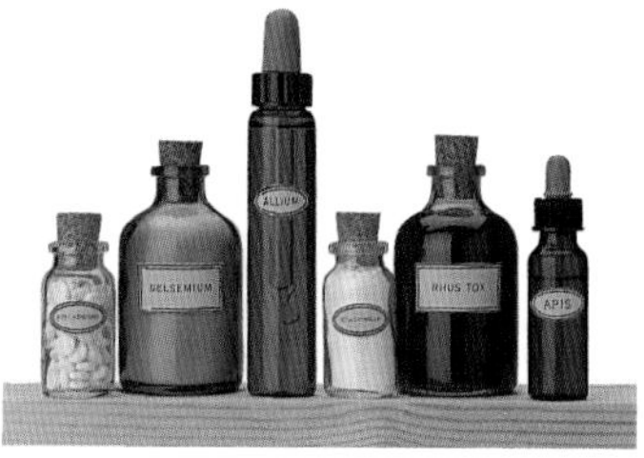

Don't worry about any symptoms listed that you don't have; the remedy only has to match the main symptoms that you do have.

Although remedies are suggested for acute flare-ups of chronic conditions such as asthma and hay fever, the remedies will only help to ease the acute symptoms. Any deep-seated chronic health problem will need treatment from an experienced professional *(see page 13–15)*.

GENERAL TREATMENT GUIDELINES

- Infections go through different stages so you may need different remedies as your infection develops. Choose the one that matches your symptoms now, and stick to it as long as you are getting some benefit.
- Don't take two different remedies at the same time, unless prescribed by a homeopath.
- If there is no improvement after five or six doses, you have probably chosen the wrong remedy.
- Don't worry about taking the wrong remedy – homeopathic remedies are harmless when taken for short periods of time.
- Reduce the frequency of taking the remedy once you have started to improve, and stop taking it once you feel much better in yourself. Your own body will do the rest.
- The golden rule is to stop once you feel better.

Common ailments

ACCIDENTS (*see p.27*)

ALLERGIC SKIN REACTIONS (*see p.24*)

ANXIETY (*see p.39*)

ARTHRITIS,INFLAMMATION, PAIN AND SWELLING OF THE JOINTS

- Bryonia (*pp.32–3*) – eases joint pains which are worse for movement.
- Rhus tox (*pp.48–9*) – joint pains ease off after gentle exercise.
- Pulsatilla (*pp.46–7*) – joint pains move from one joint to the other.
- Caullophyllum – where small joints of fingers and toes are affected.

ASTHMA

These remedies are for mild asthma only, while you are waiting for emergency attention.

- Ipecac – for wheezy children who cough till they vomit.

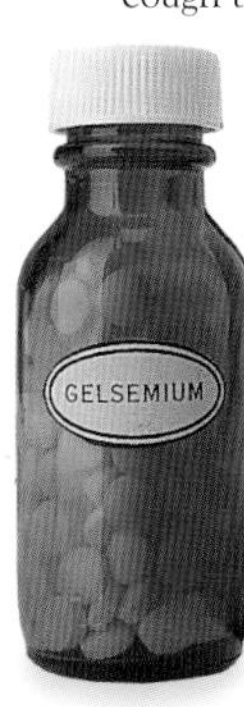

- Arsenicum (*pp.28–9*) – waking between midnight and 2 am with difficult breathing.
- Bryonia (*pp.32–3*) – asthma that comes on at the end of a cold, with a hard, dry cough.
- Natrum sulph – asthma in damp weather; loose cough, yellow mucus.
- Lachesis – asthma that comes on in spring or fall, or at the menopause.

BURNS

- Urtica urens for minor burns where the skin is blistered, and for sunburn.
- Cantharsis for more severe burns. Take the remedy in pill form as usual.

- Urtica cream can be used for minor burns, where the skin isn't broken.

COLDS

- Allium cepa – for streaming nose and eyes; nose is red raw.
- Pulsatilla (*pp.46–7*) – for runny nose with thick yellow or green mucus. Main remedy for coughing worse for lying down and on waking.
- Natrum mur – for colds with a crop of cold sores. Sneezing and watery eyes.
- Dulcamara – when nose stuffs up with catarrh in rain or wind.

See also Aconite (*pp.22–3*), Arsenicum album (*pp.28–9*), Nux vomica (*pp.42–3*), and Silica (*pp.50–51*).

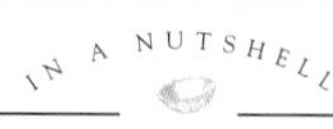

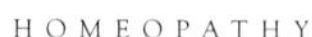

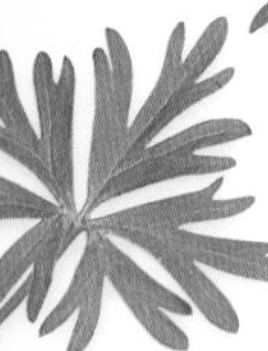

CONJUNCTIVITIS ❧

• Euphrasia – burning, watery eyes.

• One or two drops of Euphrasia tincture can also be used to bathe the eyes.

• Pulsatilla (*pp.46–7*) – conjunctivitis with mucus collecting in corner of eyes.

CONSTIPATION *(see p.33)* ❧

COUGHS ❧

• Pulsatilla (*pp.46–7*) – loose, wet, rattly cough. Worse in morning, and lying down to sleep.

• Ant tart – especially useful in elderly, who suffer from persistent rattly cough. Full of loose mucus but can't seem to bring it up.

• Rumex – very tickly cough; cold air seems to irritate nose and throat.

• Bryonia (*pp.32–3*) – for a dry cough, where the chest feels sore from coughing.

• Phosphorus (*pp.44–5*) – tickling cough in delicate people with weak chests.

CYSTITIS ❧

• Sarsaparilla – common remedy for burning pain just at the end of urinating.

• Staphysagria – known as "honeymoon cystitis," attacks are triggered off by sex.

• Nux Vomica (*pp.42–3*) – attacks from stress, or drinking lots of coffee and alcohol.

• Cantharis – intense pain, where only a few drops of urine are squeezed out.

• Pulsatilla (*pp.46–7*) – cystitis in children or pregnant women.

DENTAL PROBLEMS ❧

• Arnica (*pp.26–7*) – after dental extractions, or a lot of dental work.

• Ruta – for aching deep in the jaw after extraction if Arnica doesn't help.

• Hypericum (*pp.40–41*) – when dental work irritates the nerves, causing sharp pains.

• Ledum – where healing is poor, especially in elderly people with poor circulation. The gum feels numb and dead.

• Phosphorus (*pp.44–5*) – for easy bleeding after dental work.

DIARRHEA ❧

• Aloe – cramps just before diarrhea; and feel a bit weak after.

• Podophyllum – loose watery stool which splatters all over the bowl.

• Phosphorus (*pp.44–5*) – loose, watery diarrhea without any pain.

Feel weak and thirsty.

- Arsenicum (*pp.28–9*) – food poisoning. Diarrhea due to anxiety.

EARACHES ❧

- Aconite (*pp.22–3*) – unbearable pain in ear, with fever.
- Belladonna (*pp.30–31*) – for earache with a very high temperature.
- Chamomilla (*pp.36–7*) – for ear infections where the person is hypersensitive.
- Pulsatilla (*pp.46–7*) – for earaches which come on after a cold. Deaf from catarrh.

FAINTING ❧

- Aconite (*pp.22–3*) – sudden state of shock, causing acute panic.
- China – fainting from anemia or loss of fluids, diarrhea, or a blood transfusion.
- Ignatia – fainting from strong emotions; feels hysterical.
- Carbo veg – the body feels very cold, and the person is slow to come round.

FOOD POISONING (*see p.29*) ❧

FRACTURES ❧

After the bone has been set, homeopathic remedies help healing.

- Symphytum – from the plant called comfrey, or "bone-set." Take it daily for several weeks to help the bone knit back together.
- Calc phos – particularly good for elderly, or those with weak bones. To strengthen the bones, after the bone has knitted.

HAY FEVER ❧

These remedies will help relieve the immediate symptoms, but you will need professional treatment to cure the problem.

- Allium cepa – much sneezing and runny nose, where the mucus seems watery and burning.
- Euphrasia – where the eyes are more irritated than the nose.
- Sabadilla – constantly streaming nose with frequent bouts of violent sneezing. Sensitive to newly grown grass and the odor of flowers.
- Nux vomica (*pp.42–3*) – the main remedy for sneezing and runny nose in the morning.
- Arum triphyllum – skin below nose, and upper lip look inflamed and chapped, especially in children.

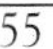

• Wyethia – very itchy roof of the mouth, when you make a funny clicking noise with the tongue.
See also Arsenicum (*pp.28–9*), Nux vomica (*pp.42–3*), and Pulsatilla (*pp.46–7*).

HEMORRHOIDS AND VARICOSE VEINS

• Hamamelis – piles tend to bleed. Hemorrhoids from pregnancy or childbirth.
• Aesculus – hemorrhoids may feel hot or burning. Sharp pains up anus.
• Pulsatilla (*pp.46–7*) – varicose veins in vulva or legs during pregnancy.

HERPES

• Natrum mur – cold sores around the lips.
• Rhus tox (*pp.48–9*) – herpes eruption on the genitals or inside of the thigh.

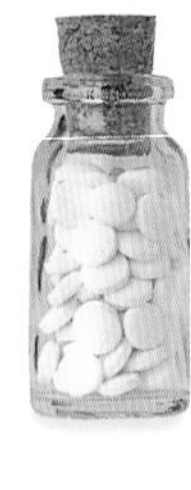

• Arsenicum (*pp.28–9*) – herpes brought on by anxiety.
• Sepia – herpes that comes on around the menstrual period.

IMPETIGO (*see p.49*)

INDIGESTION (*see p.43*)

INFLUENZA

• Gelsemium (*pp.38–9*) – muscular weakness, aching, and heaviness.
• Rhus tox (*pp.48–9*) – comes on after getting wet. There is a lot of aching in the joints rather than the muscles; restless and can't find a comfortable position.
• Bryonia (*pp.32–3*)– bad headache, and dry cough. Want to lie quite still.
• Eupatorium perfoliatum – for very intense aching in the back and limbs, with shivering chills.
• Arsenicum (*pp.28–9*) – feel debilitated, often with loss of fluids; watery diarrhea, and sometimes vomiting.
• Baptisia – for gastric flu, when very "wiped out." Body feels bruised, or scattered around the bed. Sudden bouts of diarrhea or vomiting.

INJURIES (*see p.41*)

MASTITIS (*see p.31*)

NAUSEA AND VOMITING (*see p.45*)

NOSEBLEEDS

Useful for someone who has a tendency to nosebleeds:
• Ferrum phos – during colds, nose bleeds on blowing.
• Phosphorus (*pp.44–5*) – spontaneous nosebleeds for no apparent reason.

PERIOD PROBLEMS ❧

• Belladonna (*pp.30–31*) – extremely heavy periods. Feel hot and even feverish.

• Sepia – lot of bearing down in uterus and low back pain with the period. Feel worn out and irritable. Loss of sex drive.

• Pulsatilla (*pp.46–7*) – very weepy and vulnerable before the period. Periods changeable; often both light and late.

• Nux vomica (*pp.42–3*) – bouts of rage before period.

SHINGLES (*see p.49*) ❧

SHOCK (*see p.26*) ❧

SINUSITIS ❧

• Kali bich – main remedy. Thick, sticky mucus that accumulates in the throat: difficult to clear it. Mucus gluey; looks like melted cheese, or is coughed up in strings of yellowish phlegm. Dries into sticky crusts in nose.

• Hepar sulf – try this if kali bich doesn't help.

SKIN INFECTIONS ❧

• Calendula (*pp.34–5*) – for grazes that look infected.

• Silica (*pp.50–51*) – for injuries which get infected. Swelling and pus formation around splinters or glass. Boils and abscesses.

SORE THROATS ❧

• Apis (*pp.24–5*) – especially if uvula (the sac that hangs in the middle), looks like a water blister. Sharp stinging in throat when swallowing.

• Phytolacca – glands in neck very swollen and tender. Feel fluey and achey.

• Lachesis – choke on swallowing; can't bear anything around the throat (like a collar or scarf).

• Hepar sulf – sensation of a splinter or bone stuck in the throat.

• Merc sol – when glands swollen, and body sweaty and smelly. Mouth foul and ulcerated. Tongue swollen.

• Phosphorus (*pp.44–5*) – sore throats with hoarseness or loss of voice; laryngitis. See also Aconite (*pp.22–3*) and Belladonna (*pp.30–31*).

SPRAINS ❧

• Rhus tox (poison ivy) (*pp.48–9*) – aching that persists and gets worse in damp weather. The joint is stiff in the

morning, and only limbers up after exercise.

- Ruta – if Rhus tox hasn't helped after five or six days.

STYES ❧

- Staphysagria – after a period of bottling up anger and resentment
- Pulsatilla (*pp.46–7*)– styes when run down or after a cold; yellow pus in the corner of the eye.

TEETHING ❧

- Chamomilla (*pp.36–7*) – available as teething granules for fractious teething children. The remedy can also help toothache in adults. The pain is worse for breathing in cold air and drinking coffee or anything cold.

THRUSH ❧

- Pulsatilla (*pp.46–7*) – thick creamy or yellowish discharge, may not be very irritating.
- Borax – discharge looks more like egg white; can feel it running out.

TOOTHACHE ❧

- Ferrum phos – for mild toothache, only on exposure to heat and cold.
- Belladonna (*pp.30–31*) – if the pain comes on exposure to heat and cold.
- Chamomilla (*pp.36–7*) – helps relieve unbearable pain.
- Staphysagria – for toothache from cold drinks. Psychologically resentful; dental work is intrusive.
- Nux vomica (*pp.42–3*) – if you feel oversensitive to pain, irritable and bad tempered.
- Plantago – toothache in badly decayed teeth.
- Cheiranthus – for swelling or infection around the wisdom teeth.

TRAVEL SICKNESS ❧

- Cocculus – sick and dizzy. Want to lie down. The thought of food makes sickness worse.
- Tabaccum – pale and sweaty with the nausea. Feel cold but need fresh air. Can't tolerate cigarette smoke.

WARTS ❧

- Thuja – for warts on the face, or crops of veruccas.
- Causticum – warts on the nose, or around the fingernails.
- Nitric acid – warts round the anus.
- Thuja tincture can be applied daily to veruccas. Buy it in a dropper bottle, and use it undiluted.

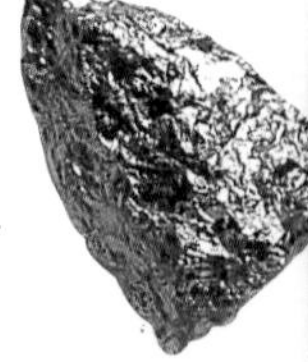

WOUNDS (see *p.35*) ❧

Further reading

Dr. Christopher Hammond, THE COMPLETE FAMILY GUIDE TO HOMEOPATHY (Element Books, 1995)

Robin Hayfield, HOMEOPATHY, A PRACTICAL GUIDE TO EVERYDAY HEALTHCARE (Gaia Books, 1994)

Dana Ullman, HOMEOPATHY: MEDICINE FOR THE 21ST CENTURY (Thorsons, 1988)

George Vithoulkas, HOMEOPATHY; MEDICINE FOR THE NEW MAN (Thorsons, 1985)

Useful addresses

SUPPLIERS

Ainsworths Homeopathic Pharmacy
36 New Cavendish Street
London W1M 7LH
Tel: 020 7935 5330

Nelson's Homeopathic Pharmacy
73 Duke Street
London W1K 5BY
Tel: 020 7629 3118

Helios Homeopathic Pharmacy
97 Camden Road
Tunbridge Wells
Kent TN1 2QR
Tel: 01892 537254

Galen Homeopathics
Llewell, Dorchester
Dorset DT2 8AN
Tel: 01305 263996

American Association of Homeopathic Pharmacies
3741 Mitford Lane
Clinton WA 98236 USA

SOCIETIES AND ASSOCIATIONS

British Homeopathic Association
15 Clerkenwell Close
London EC1R 0AA
Tel: 020 7566 7800

New York Homeopathic Medical Society
110–156 71st Avenue, Ste 1-H
Forest Hills
NY 11371 USA

ALTERNATIVE TREATMENT CENTERS

The British Homeopathic Dental Association
15 Clerkenwell Close
London EC1R 0AA
Tel: 020 7566 7800

The British Association of Homeopathic Chiropodists
15 Clerkenwell Close
London EC1R 0AA
Tel: 020 7566 7800